D0258593

Evidence-based Practice in Primary Care
Second edition

Evidence-based Practice in Primary Care

Second edition

Edited by
Chris Silagy

Professor and Director, Institute of Health Services Research,
Monash University, Australia

and

Andrew Haines

Professor of Public Health and Primary Care and Dean, London School
of Hygiene and Tropical Medicine, London, UK

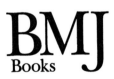

BMJ
Books

© BMJ Books 2001
BMJ Books is an imprint of the BMJ Publishing Group

First published in 1998
Reprinted 1999
Second edition 2001
by BMJ Books, BMA House, Tavistock Square,
London WC1H 9JR

www.bmjbooks.com

British Library Cataloguing in Publication Data

A catalogue record for this book is available from the British Library

ISBN 0 7279 1568 1

Contents

Contributors

Baker R, Clinical Governance Research and Development Unit, Department of General Practice and Primary Health Care, University of Leicester, UK

Cumbers B, Library, Central Middlesex Hospital NHS Trust, London, UK

Davis D, Office of Continuing Education, Faculty of Medicine, University of Toronto, Canada

Del Mar C, Centre for General Practice, University of Queensland Medical School, Australia

Eccles M, Centre for Health Services Research, University of Newcastle upon Tyne, UK

Flottorp S, Health Services Research Unit, National Institute of Public Health, Oslo, Norway

Gill P, Department of Primary Care and General Practice, University of Birmingham, UK

Greenhalgh T, Department of Primary Care and Population Sciences, Royal Free and University College Medical School, London, UK

Grimshaw J, Health Services Research Unit, University of Aberdeen, UK

Grol R, Centre for Quality of Care Research, Universities of Nijmegen and Maastricht, The Netherlands

Haines A, London School of Hygiene and Tropical Medicine, London, UK

Kidd M, Department of General Practice, The University of Sydney, Australia

Knottnerus JA, Netherlands School of Primary Care Research, University of Maastricht, The Netherlands

Lancaster T, Department of Primary Health Care, Oxford University, Oxford, UK

Lloyd M, Department of Primary Care and Population Sciences, Royal Free and University College Medical School, London, UK

O'Brien MA, Chedoke–McMaster Hospitals, Hamilton, Canada

Oxman A, Health Services Research Unit, National Institute of Public Health, Oslo, Norway

Purves I, Sowerby Centre for Health Informatics, University of Newcastle upon Tyne, UK

Rogers S, Department of Primary Care and Population Sciences, Royal Free and University College Medical School, London, UK

Silagy CA, Institute of Health Services Research, Monash University, Australia

Weingarten M, Department of Family Medicine, Sackler School of Medicine, Tel Aviv University, Israel

Weller D, Department of General Practice, University of Edinburgh, Edinburgh, UK

Wentz R, Imperial College Library, Chelsea and Westminster Hospital, London, UK

Winkens RAG, Transmural and Diagnostic Centre, Maastricht, The Netherlands

Young G, The Surgery, Barn Croft, Temple Sowerby, Penrith, Cumbria, UK

Preface to the second edition

During the last decade, the concepts of evidence-based practice have stimulated wide-ranging interest amongst health professionals as one of the central foundations underpinning the organisation and provision of health care services. Some people have suggested evidence-based practice represents a new paradigm whilst others argue it is nothing more than a repackaging of old concepts wrapped in new jargon. Irrespective of these divergent views, there is little doubt that the ideas embraced by evidence-based practice are beginning to impact on most health care disciplines, including general practice.

Although there are other books on various aspects of evidence-based practice, many of these have focused on the acquisition of specific skills, such as critical appraisal, or on the wide implications for the health system of systematically using research evidence to influence health policy and practice. However, there has been a paucity of information targeting the relevance of evidence-based approaches specifically to general practice. General practice is, by its very nature, a highly complex discipline that has been characterised by a high proportion of less well-differentiated problems that frequently highlight the interplay between biological, psychological and social factors. Through trying to confront and unravel these factors, we became increasingly aware of the need for a book which specifically addressed the relevance and place of evidence-based practice for primary care practitioners. We have elected to use the term "general practitioner" although we are, of course, aware of the different terminology employed to describe primary care doctors around the world. In addition, we recognise the importance of a multidisciplinary approach to involving the primary care team in activities to promote effective practice.

This book is not intended to be a step by step "how to do it" guide. For general practitioners who are interested in developing a detailed knowledge and skills in this area, a list of further reading and other resources is provided. There are also a growing number of short courses on evidence-based practice which are being offered by academic institutions and professional societies throughout the world. Instead, it informs those general practitioners and primary care teams who wish to gain an *overview* of the topic.

The book is organised into two separate parts. The first deals with the approach to utilising an evidence-based approach to the care of individual patients. It begins with how to ask and refine a good clinical question, then track down the necessary evidence and critically appraise it. Subsequent chapters deal with how to apply the evidence, the latter of the two having a specific focus on the application of evidence relating to screening and diagnostic tests. The final chapter in Part 1 deals with how to evaluate the impact of applying the evidence. In the second part of the book, the focus is on the strategies required at professional and disciplinary level in order to develop an ongoing culture of evidence-based practice within primary care. These include clinical practice guidelines, use of computerised decision support systems and continuing medical education strategies.

Contributors have been drawn from six countries. This is reflected in the diversity of writing styles and examples which are used to illustrate the relevance of evidence-based health care to general practice throughout the world. The experience of the contributors is largely in primary medical care in industrialised countries but the underlying concepts discussed are also relevant to primary care in other nations. Some topics, such as the performance of diagnostic and screening tests, are covered more than once in the book at different levels of detail. We have allowed them to remain in the text so that individual chapters are complete in themselves, but have cross referenced where relevant to other chapters.

The success of the first edition prompted us to prepare this second edition. We wish to thank all the contributors for their patience and cooperation in complying with our requests for revisions and rewrites, Drs Trisha Greenhalgh, Paul Glasziou, Linda Geron, Anita Berlin, and Jane Russell who kindly reviewed parts of the manuscript and provided extremely helpful comments and suggestions which greatly improved the end product; Ms C O'Connor and Ms R Burnley who assisted in the final preparation of the manuscripts; and Ms Mary Banks from BMJ Books who provided support and encouragement throughout the preparation of the book. Finally, we also wish to thank our respective families for their tolerance and patience when the time that should have been theirs was spent preparing this book.

Chris Silagy and Andrew Haines

1: Evidence-based practice in primary care: an introduction

CHRIS SILAGY AND DAVID WELLER

Introduction

This book aims to explore the concept of evidence-based practice (EBP) in terms of its relevance and applicability to general practice. We recognise that neither is EBP a new concept, nor is its application in general practice a straightforward task. Indeed, some argue that the culture of EBP is too narrow and overly prescriptive to be made relevant to the complexities and uncertainty of general practice.

The task of this book is not to dismiss potential barriers to applying EBP in general practice, but rather to examine methods of integrating and promoting the uptake of EBP in such a way that it takes account of the complexities of the discipline. Indeed, with the growing demand for public accountability in health care and the increased availability of information to users of health care services, it is likely that EBP will be a central theme in general practice and the organisation of care for many years to come.

The need for an evidence-based approach to decision-making in general practice

The core of general practice is the relationship between the doctor and patient.[1] One of the central aspects of this relationship is the process of decision-making, which can range from the simple clinical types of decision (this patient has a sore throat; it's red but there is no pus – should antibiotics be prescribed?, or, this patient has complained of frontal headaches, for two weeks, which are present on waking – should a CT scan be carried out?) to decisions at a practice level about how services should be organised (for example, is the establishment of a specialised, multidisciplinary mini-clinic within the practice likely to result in improved care for diabetic patients?). In each case, the decisions ought to involve a negotiated arrangement which occurs in the context of a partnership between the health care professional and patient (or between the team of primary health care professionals and their practice population), and takes account of factors such as patient need, preferences, priorities, available resources and evidence of the effects of providing different forms of care (Figure 1.1).

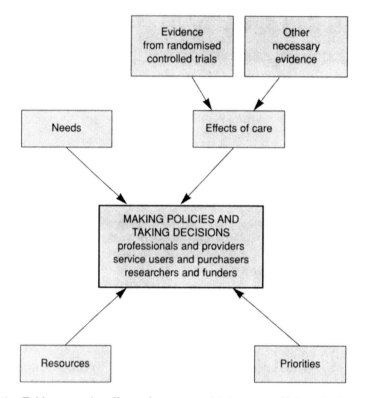

Fig 1.1 Evidence on the effects of care: essential, but not sufficient, for improving policies and decisions in health care and research. (Cochrane Collaboration brochure 1995.)

Both the doctor and patient require access to reliable and valid information about each of these factors, which they can then consider applying to the situation where a decision is required. Evidence based medicine is the phrase used to describe such an approach and entails (from the doctor's perspective) "the conscientious, explicit and judicious use of current best evidence in making decisions about the care of individual patients".[2]

Evidence based health care has never been promoted as a total substitute for clinical experience. General practitioners acquire proficiency, wisdom and judgement through their clinical experience; this expertise produces clinical skill and acumen in detecting physical signs and symptoms, as well as a greater understanding of individuals' "predicaments, rights and preferences in making clinical decisions about their care". Clinical experience is therefore an important component of decision-making in general practice as it is the means by which research evidence can be put in context and individualised to specific clinical encounters. On the other hand, overreliance on clinical experience can be misleading, giving rise to false impressions of the benefit or harm from interventions.[3]

Many general practitioners would argue that they have always tried to take account of evidence when making clinical decisions, and find it difficult to understand what all the fuss is about with the recent emergence of interest in evidence-based medicine. In responding to this view, it is important to emphasise that evidence-based approaches build on and support, rather than directly challenge, the traditional values of health care practice. In particular, there have been a number of developments during the past few decades which make it much easier to adopt an evidence-based approach to health care decision-making.[4] These include the availability of better research methods for assessing the validity of evidence of effectiveness through to improved techniques for collating evidence in a systematic way. These changes have been accompanied by a gradual shift within health care from an authoritarian culture to a more authoritative culture. This shift has occurred as a direct result of placing greater *emphasis* and value on the doctor's ability to access and appropriately use knowledge rather than on any historical position of power and influence.

The distinction between evidence-based medicine and evidence-based health care

It is useful to distinguish at this point the difference between the terms evidence-based medicine and evidence-based health care (EBHC). The former is a conceptual approach that health care professionals (particularly doctors) can use in making decisions about the care of individual patients. By contrast, EBHC is a somewhat broader concept that incorporates improved approaches to understanding patients', families' and practitioners' beliefs, values and attitudes (often through qualitative research methods). EBHC also takes account of evidence at a population level (such as the burden of disease and implications for resource utilisation) as well as encompassing interventions concerned with the organisation and delivery of health care (including that provided by health care professionals other than doctors). There is little value in debating whether there is a clear line to divide the two approaches, and for the purposes of this book we have decided to focus on the broader definition of EBHC since it encompasses the general practitioner's responsibility to their practice population as well as to individual patients. To avoid conflict relating to terminology we have chosen to use a more neutral term, evidence-based practice (EBP), throughout the text. This terminology also highlights the use of evidence both in individual patient care and in the organisation of services for the practice population.

The gap between research and practice

One of the major reasons why there has been so much interest in evidence-based approaches to health care is the growing number of examples where current medical practice has lagged significantly behind the available research evidence. For example, despite strong evidence during the 1970s that treatments such as thrombolytic therapy and aspirin were effective in the treatment of acute myocardial infarction, it took almost a further decade before these treatments were being recommended routinely.[5] Similarly, there are examples of widely (and sometimes excessively) used practices, such as dilatation and curettage for dysfunctional uterine bleeding, where for a number of years there has been evidence of lack of effectiveness.[5] The reason for this apparent gap between the available scientific research evidence and its application in practice is complex. In some instances, it reflects upon the lack of rigour which has been applied to synthesising results of primary research in a systematic manner. In other instances, it reflects the inability of the available research evidence to provide the relevant information that consumers and health care professionals need to make decisions. At a broader level, it reflects upon the lack of appropriate frameworks, systems and strategies for effectively influencing professional behaviour.

The complexity of general practice

It is widely acknowledged that skills necessary for general practice go well beyond diagnosis and treatment of illness; other important elements include aspects of sociology, pastoral care, or even mythology. Patients present in general practice with multiple and ill-defined problems – single, discrete problems are rare. As a result, general practitioners are often faced with difficulty in identifying a clear diagnosis and formulating an explicit plan of management. More often than not there will be unanswered questions following a consultation; some issues will be addressed immediately, others will require time to either develop or resolve. The complex nature of general practice means that often individuals seek help in aspects of illness for which there may be no convincing evidence of the effectiveness of any intervention.[6]

This complexity and lack of evidence should not be seen as a reason for jettisoning the use of evidence in those areas where it does exist, and is an argument for continually seeking to develop and refine our capacity to collect new evidence, in a rigorous manner, in those areas where it does not exist. In fact, a report by Gill *et al.*,[7] based on a retrospective analysis of a consecutive series of doctor–patient encounters, found that a high proportion (81%) of interventions in general practice could be supported by evidence from randomised controlled trials and/or convincing nonexperimental evidence. Although there have been methodological criticisms of the study, it does highlight the potential of using evidence to inform a considerable proportion of decision-making in general practice.

There is still a need to refine how evidence can be incorporated into the complexity of the doctor–patient relationship in general practice. For example, currently a major research effort is being undertaken to develop methods of incorporating the weighted preferences of patients into models of decision analysis.[8] This may ultimately represent an important advance in creating a useful resource for decision-making in general practice. As we begin to understand more about the contribution of other aspects of the decision-making process, such as the importance of information sharing and the ethical values held by the doctor and patient, it is likely that methodologies for understanding and applying an evidence-based approach will continue to be refined and improved.

How to get started: a five-step process for using an evidence-based approach in general practice

How should busy general practitioners get started if they want to embrace an evidence-based approach as part of their practice? The McMaster University Evidence Based Medicine Resource Group have identified a five-step approach that individual health care professionals need to follow:[9]

(1) define the problem;
(2) track down the information sources you need;
(3) critically appraise the information;
(4) apply the information with your patients;
(5) evaluate how effective this application of information is.

These five steps are reviewed briefly in this chapter and discussed in more detail in later chapters.

Step 1: defining the problem

In every consultation decisions need to be made. Many of these are done almost subconsciously, with little or no formal critical evaluation. Questions frequently arise, such as the pros and cons of using a particular form of therapy, the value of having a particular diagnostic test or screening procedure, the risk or prognosis of a particular disease, or the cost (and cost-effectiveness) of a potential intervention. Rather than relying solely on our memories to answer such questions (which may not represent the most up-to-date summary of the available clinical information), an evidence-based approach would be to pause and recognise that there is a clinical problem for which you are unsure of the evidence and to make a decision to investigate it further.

Clearly, it is not possible within a busy general practice to embark on a detailed search of the scientific evidence for every question that arises. Establishing a system for prioritising and refining questions will be addressed in Chapter 2.

Step 2: tracking down the information sources needed

General practitioners face difficulties above and beyond their specialist colleagues in gaining access to research findings.[10] The body of medical literature which can assist in providing answers to the questions raised in clinical practice is broadly scattered; journals of ear, nose and throat or mental health, specialist general practice and family medicine journals and government reports all contain information which may be of relevance. The challenge (which is discussed further in Chapter 3) is to identify what is available and accessible through a variety of means, including searching electronic databases, consulting research synthesis journals and communicating with colleagues. An increasingly common scenario that can facilitate tracking down relevant information involves patients arriving at the surgery having completed literature searches of their own.

Step 3: critically appraising the information

Having decided which journal articles to read, it is important to read them carefully as not all published information is of equal value. Critical appraisal of articles is a process which involves carefully reading an article and analysing its methodology, content, and conclusions. The key question to keep in mind is: "Do I believe these results sufficiently that I would be prepared to adopt a similar approach, or reach a similar conclusion, with my own patients?"

The skill of being able to critically appraise articles needs to be learned and practised like any other clinical skill. There are a range of different approaches to critical appraisal, depending on the type of question being asked; this will be addressed further in Chapter 4.

Step 4: applying the information with your patients

The fourth step in the process of using an evidence-based approach to the practice of health care is to decide how to apply the information obtained to the particular circumstances of your patient. This is probably the most crucial step in the process, as well as the most complex, and will be examined in detail in Chapters 5 and 6.

It is necessary to decide whether there are any methodological issues raised about the evidence which might prompt you to reject it outright. Assuming there are no such issues involved, there is a need to assess the trade-offs between any adverse and beneficial effects as well as decide how to take into account an assessment of the patient's stated (and perceived) needs, the resources available and the priorities that may be placed by the patient on different treatment options. This process requires a partnership between the doctor and patient. If at the end of that process the decision is made not to apply the available research evidence, that decision should be a mutual and conscious one.

Step 5: evaluating how effective it is

The final step in using an evidence-based approach (which is discussed in Chapter 7) is to evaluate the effect of the evidence as applied to specific patients. This is an important step in "closing the loop", to gauge whether the expected benefits that arose from using a particular item of evidence were consistent with the observed benefits. If the observed benefits are less than had been expected from the evidence, it may well generate the need for further research to identify why some patients have not responded in the expected manner and what can be done to rectify this.

There is nothing particularly conceptually difficult about these five steps; they can be readily taught at an undergraduate level and then reinforced at a postgraduate level. The practical problem in the "real world" facing busy general practitioners is having sufficient time to apply these steps routinely in their daily practice.

Supporting a framework for evidence-based practice within general practice

The second part of this book describes the challenges and responsibilities facing general practitioners as professionals that need to be addressed if an evidence-based approach is to flourish. Such a framework needs to be built around ensuring that the evidence required to inform decision-making is available, accessible, acceptable and applied by general practitioners, as well as putting in place strategies to thoroughly evaluate the impact of applying the evidence. For example, there is an overwhelming amount of research evidence available, with over two million new articles added to the world's medical literature each year.[11] Even in the primary care literature there are probably now five times as many randomised controlled trials as there were about 20 years ago.[12] Keeping up to date with all of this is a daunting task, particularly since the evidence (even when limited to a single discipline) is published across a wide range of journals and is of variable quality and relevance. General practitioners have little hope of coming to grips with this body of material unassisted – they lack time and often do not have access to the necessary skills or resources to undertake searching, critical appraisal and assessment of relevance to general practice.

Several initiatives have recently emerged internationally which aim to produce systematic summaries of literature, thereby relieving a great deal of the burden associated with trying to practise EBP. Good examples are the Cochrane Library (a database of high quality systematic reviews covering all fields of health care, including general practice) and the journals of secondary publication, such as the AGP Journal Club, Evidence Based Medicine and Clinical Evidence, which undertake the task of scanning the medical literature and compiling summary commentaries together with structured abstracts on particular topics, after a process of critical appraisal and quality assessment of material (see Appendix 2, p 190 for further details).

At a more local level, there are a growing number of networks being established around the world amongst general practitioners who wish to share the tasks of searching for and appraising evidence.[13] Some of these networks meet face to face whilst others concentrate on electronic media for communicating. Support mechanisms such as these can allow busy clinicians to devote their scarce reading time to "selective, efficient, patient-driven searching," and incorporation of the best available evidence in order to practise evidence-based health care.

A natural extension of this process is to apply evidence-based protocols and guidelines, developed by our colleagues, in clinical practice. Systematic reviews may provide a sound basis for the development of clinical guidelines.

Two other important features of evidence which affect whether it is likely to be implemented in clinical practice are its acceptability and applicability. There is little value in gaining access to evidence if it is not relevant to the GP's patients, or if the health intervention it examines is not acceptable or available in a particular practice setting. In the absence of these features which are discussed further in Chapter 8, exposure to evidence from the literature is likely to have little effect on clinical practice.

To examine the question of whether exposure to research evidence can change practice behaviour, Oxman *et al.* reviewed 102 randomised controlled trials in which changes in physician behaviour were attempted through means such as continuing medical education workshops and seminars, educational materials, academic detailing and audit and feedback.[14] Each produced some change, but the authors concluded that a multifaceted strategy was called for, using combinations of methods.

Chapter 9 examines the specific role of clinical practice guidelines in supporting clinical decision-making; Chapters 10 and 11 discuss the role of information technology and continuing education respectively in helping practitioners keep up to date with the sheer volume and rapidly changing knowledge base, while Chapter 12 discusses factors affecting the integration of evidence into practice via these and other methods that are used to promote change.

There is growing interest in individualising the results of research evidence and developing co-ordinated strategies which can take into account factors such as the strength of evidence, methodological limitations, relative trade-offs between adverse and beneficial effects (after adjustment for patient's baseline risks) as well as evidence of patient beliefs, attitudes and values.[15]

Finally, there must be the capacity to evaluate the uptake of EBP in general practice. Critics of EBP in general practice often argue that uptake of evidence-based health practises is difficult or impossible to evaluate. Why promote the concept of EBP if we can never be sure that decision-making in general practice has been influenced by the process? (as discussed in Chapter 7). In theory, evidence-based health practises should lead to improvements in health outcomes, but not all general practice interventions can be linked directly to health outcomes. Furthermore, in many aspects of health care there are long lag times; for example, in cancer or cardiovascular disease, the time between the GP's health interventions and any measurable outcomes may be considerable. There is a concern that a strong adherence to EBP may lead to a focus on those health interventions in general practice for which outcomes are easily and immediately measured.

Other than measurable health outcomes, there are a number of proxy measures which can be used to establish whether or not health care in general practice is evidence-based. These include case-note audit for process measures, level of usage of evidence-based clinical practice guidelines and access to decision support systems. Furthermore, widespread adoption of EBP in general practice should lead to measurable reductions in variability between GPs, practices, or geographical regions in areas such as prescribing and ordering of investigations.[16] Monitoring such changes is complex and requires highly specialised systems that are capable of tracking large amounts of data on patients across different health care sectors. Developing such systems will need to be an important priority in the future development of EBP.

Summary

In this chapter we have described what EBP is, how it is applied to general practice, and what frameworks are required if general practitioners (as individuals) and general practice (as a discipline) are to embrace the concept.

We contend that if the concept is embraced it will improve general practice in a number of different ways. Firstly, it will make general practice an even more rewarding discipline within which to practice.[13] Secondly, it will support shared decision-making with users, which is increasingly advocated as the ideal model of making decisions within the medical encounter.[17] Finally, EBP will help maintain the central role of general practice in health care.[18] In an environment with an increasing focus on both the accountability of health expenditure and identification and measurement of health outcomes for all health interventions, it would be perilous to ignore EBP in general practice.

References

1 Heath I. *The mystery of general practice.* London: Nuffield Provincial Hospitals Trust, 1995.
2 Sackett D, Rosenberg WMC, Gray JAM, *et al.* Evidence based medicine: what it is and what it isn't. *BMJ* 1996;**313**:169–71.
3 Antman EM, Lau J, Kupelnick B, *et al.* A comparison of the results of meta-analyses of randomised control trials and recommendations of clinical experts. Treatments for myocardial infarction. *JAMA* 1992;**268**:240–8.
4 Evidence Based Medicine Working Group. Evidence based medicine. A new approach to teaching the practice of medicine. *JAMA* 1992;**268**:2420–5.
5 Coulter A. Diagnostic dilation and curettage: is it used appropriately? *BMJ* 1993;**306**(6872): 236–9.
6 Greenhalgh T. Is my practice evidence-based? *BMJ* 1996;**313**(7063):957–8.
7 Gill P, Dowell AC, Neal RD, Smith N, Heywood P, Wilson AR. Evidence based general practice: a retrospective study of interventions in one training practice. *BMJ* 1996;**312**:819–21.
8 Blaxter M. *Consumers and research in NHS: consumer issues within the NHS.* Report no. G60/002 2954. Leeds: Department of Health Publications, 1994.
9 Sackett DL, Richardson WS, Rosenberg W, Haynes RB. *Evidence-based medicine: how to practise and teach EBM.* London: Churchill Livingstone, 1997.
10 Haines A, Jones R. Implementing findings of research. *BMJ* 1994;**308**:1488–92.
11 Mulrow CD. Rationale for systematic reviews. In: Chalmers I, Altman DG, eds. *Systematic reviews.* London: BMJ Publishing Group, 1995.
12 Silagy C. Developing a register of randomised controlled trials in primary care. *BMJ* 1993;**306**:897–900.
13 Dawes M. On the need for evidence-based general and family practice. *Evidence Based Med* 1996;1:68–9.
14 Oxman A, Thornson MA, Davis DA, Haynes RB. No magic bullets: a systematic review of 102 trials of interventions to improve professional practice. *Can Med Assoc J* 1995;**153**:1423–31.
15 Glasziou P, Irwig L. An evidence-based approach to individualising treatment. *BMJ* 1995;**311**:1356–9.
16 Henry D, O'Connell D. *Variability on prescribing of pharmaceuticals by general practitioners and factors related to the variability.* Australian Institute of Health and Welfare, 1996.
17 Charles C, Gafni A, Whelan T. Shared decision-making in the medical

encounter: what does it mean (or it takes at least two to tango). *Soc Sci Med* 1997;**44**:681–92.

18 Baker M, Maskrey N, Kirk S. *Clinical effectiveness and primary care.* Abingdon: Radcliffe Medical Press, 1997.

Part 1 – Evidence-based health care and the individual patient

2: Getting started: how to set priorities and define questions

PARAMJIT GILL AND MARGARET LLOYD

Introduction

Individuals bring problems to their general practitioner which tend to be multiple, diverse in nature, and which do not always signify the presence of disease. These problems need to be elicited, defined and managed appropriately. General practitioners are generalists who "unpack these undifferentiated problems" into diagnoses which may need to be referred to the secondary sector for further refinement and management. Medical students are taught to gather and use all the information about a patient (history, clinical examination and investigations) in order to make a diagnosis; this is called the inductive method of decision-making. General practitioners tend to use a different method which involves gathering information from the patient, formulating a hypothesis to explain their presenting problem and then gathering further information in order to prove or refute that hypothesis; this is called the hypothetico–deductive method and is illustrated in Figure 2.1.[1]

Many factors related to the patient, the doctor and the practice influence decision-making in general practice (Figure 2.2). We use different sorts of knowledge and clinical information culled from many sources to help to reach decisions. It is important to realise when our clinical experience is sufficient and when something more than experience is required. How can the evidence-based approach be used by the primary care team when time is limited? In this chapter we look at how to use it by defining the questions which need to be answered. During a surgery session a general practitioner will see patients with a wide range of common problems such as those shown in Box 2.1. How can we ensure that we are providing the patient with the most clinically effective care? In Chapter 1, the gap which exists between evidence and clinical practice was illustrated and how to access research evidence will be discussed in Chapter 3. The problem is that limited time does not allow us to attempt to access the evidence for every problem a patient presents and it will not

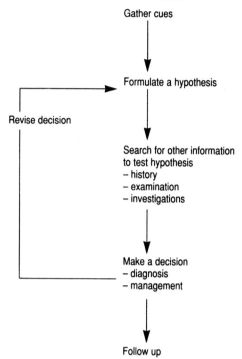

Fig 2.1 The hypothetico-deductive method of decision-making. (Based on model described by McWhinney.[1])

Box 2.1 How should these patients be managed?

- Mrs C, aged 59 years, cellulitis following an insect bite on forearm
- Mrs D, aged 73 years, feeling tired, blood pressure 200/90
- Daniel S, aged 5 years, difficulty in hearing his teacher at school, has fluid in middle ear
- Mrs K, aged 63 years, feeling "low" and tired, husband died last week
- Mr W, aged 81 years, insomnia, asks "does melatonin work?"
- Mr X, aged 31 years, chronic low back pain, asks to be referred to a chiropractor
- Mr V, aged 39 years, complains of indigestion

---

always be necessary. For example, considering the management of the patients illustrated in Box 2.1:

- Mrs C's cellulitis will almost certainly respond to flucloxacillin. Penicillin was never subjected to clinical trials before being widely used – empirical observation was enough and our own clinical experience confirms this.
- Mrs D is an elderly patient with systolic hypertension. To treat or not to

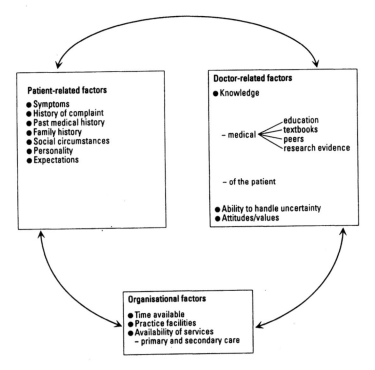

Fig 2.2 Factors influencing decision-making in general practice

treat? A number of guidelines on the management of hypertension in the elderly have been published[2] and would prove helpful. However, as will be discussed in Chapter 8, it is important that guidelines are evidence-based and that the patient's preference is taken into account when interpreting them (as discussed in Chapter 5).

- Systematic reviews of research evidence are available for a number of conditions including glue ear,[3] and reference to these would guide the management of Daniel S.
- Mrs K, who was recently bereaved, needs a listening ear and appropriate support. We do not need evidence from empirical research to provide her with effective care, although what we do can be informed by evidence of a different kind derived from the recording and interpretation of people's experience.[4] If Mrs K has an abnormal bereavement reaction then we may find that reference to a systematic review of intervention trials is helpful.[5]

This leaves a number of problems which you may think research evidence will help you to solve but, as your time is limited, how do you decide which to tackle first?

Setting priorities

Having decided to adopt an evidence-based approach to practice, asking the following questions may help you to set your priorities:[6]

- Is the problem commonly seen in practice?
- Does it have important consequences?
- What are the potential benefits of treatment?
- What are the potential risks?
- What are the costs?

Not all questions need to be answered now and by yourself. Selection of the question you wish to pursue, using the evidence-based approach, will depend on the importance it holds for you and your practice. The criteria you use may include, for example, the frequency and severity of the problem in your practice, the implication for your prescribing, or referral patterns. These may be related to the priorities above.

Considering the patients in Box 2.1 and using the above criteria, it can be argued that the problem of the management of systolic hypertension, presented by Mrs D, would be judged the top priority. However, Mr W's question about the use of melatonin in the management of insomnia and your reading of a recently published article[7] might have fired your enthusiasm for exploring the evidence-based approach to patient management.

Formulating a question

The first stage in the evidence-based approach is to ask a question which is potentially answerable (see Chapter 1). Of course, as general practitioners, we are continually asking questions during each patient encounter. Should I refer this patient to hospital? What tests do I need to do? Which hypotensive drug should I prescribe for this elderly patient? However, when using the evidence-based approach the question needs to be as focused as possible. The formulation of the question is a fundamental and challenging part of using this approach and it is important to spend some time on this as the next stage – searching for the evidence – will become much easier. We can illustrate this by considering Mr V's problem of indigestion:

Mr V has had indigestion for a number of years and it is usually helped by the ranitidine tablets he always carries with him during his business trips abroad. However, his latest attack whilst he was in India was particularly bad and lasted longer than usual. He attributed this to the stress he was under in his business but because his symptoms were not responding to ranitidine he decided to consult his general practitioner.

What questions does this scenario stimulate you to ask? You may have included some of the following questions in your list.

- What is the likely cause of his indigestion?
- What diagnostic tests would be useful?
- What reliability and validity do these tests have, particularly the test for Helicobacterpylori (*H. pylori*)?
- If Mr V does have *H. pylori* infection, what is the most cost-effective treatment?
- What is his prognosis if he is treated?
- What is his prognosis if he is not treated?
- Can we prevent the occurrence of disease by screening for *H. pylori*?

All the above questions are important but still not focused enough. It is essential to make the question specific to the patient's problem. Sackett *et al.*[8] provide a framework which helps us to build answerable questions (Table 2.1). The four-part framework includes the type of patient or problem, the intervention and comparison (if appropriate) and the outcome of interest. For example, if Mr V is confirmed to have *H. pylori* infection then we may want to know what can be done about it with drugs. The question can then be formulated, as shown in Table 2.1. Mr V may have a different question which he wants answered and this may require a different type of evidence as discussed in Chapter 5.

Table 2.1 How to build a question

	Patient or problem	Intervention	Comparison intervention	Outcome
Tips for building	Starting with your patient, ask "How would I describe a group of patients similar to mine?"	Ask "Which main intervention am I considering?"	Ask "What is the main alternative to compare with the intervention?"	Ask "What can I hope to accomplish?"
Example	*In a 39-year-old man ...*	*...does the addition of antibiotics ...*	*...compared with no antibiotics ...*	*...lead to the eradication of H. pylori and for how long?*

If you are having problems stating the question as described, write it down using the headings from Table 2.1 and look at each component separately. Try to focus your thinking on specifying clearly what you want to know. Better still, get together with a colleague(s) from your practice or elsewhere and discuss each other's questions. This will also ensure that the question is important and worth answering not only for you but for the whole practice (see above: Setting priorities). This skill of formulating a question can be practised anytime and anywhere, for example, at the end of the consultation, on the way back from a home visit, or on the bus! You just have to remember the four components.

Because time is limited it may be necessary to prioritise the questions posed by a particular patient.

What kind of research evidence?

When we embark on research the appropriate methodology is adopted to answer the research question. The same principle applies in practising evidence-based health care; the appropriate evidence, quantitative or qualitative, is located to answer the specific question. Much of the work within general practice consists of medicine that combines science with clinical judgement; in addition to the "scientific evidence" verbal and non-verbal information obtained from a patient consulting about a problem, the doctor's knowledge of the patient's psychosocial background and clinical experience of the doctor obtained by discussion with colleagues are also important.[9]

An evidence-based approach is more than using the results of randomised trials and meta-analyses; it involves locating the best external evidence to answer a clinical problem.[10] This evidence can arise from either quantitative or qualitative research. For example, you may want to know if the age and sex of patients contribute to variations in prescribing costs between practices and why do general practitioners adopt new drugs? The first question is answered by a quantitative study[11] and the second by a qualitative design.[12] This is why question formulation needs thought before searching for the answers.

Applying research evidence in general practice

Much of the available evidence is based in the secondary care sector where specialists manage specific diagnoses and problems (Figure 2.3). Not only is this evidence, including randomised trials, undertaken in the secondary sector but it then is applied to the general practice setting.[13] This raises problems of generalisability and how results of a study apply to a particular patient in a particular practice (see Chapter 5). Furthermore, the *emphasis* has been on the quantitative aspects of diagnosis and management and not the qualitative features which are essential to general practice.[14]

Finding research evidence

Many of these potentially answerable questions cannot be answered as the evidence will not be found.[15] This does not devalue the process of asking questions; it highlights the knowledge gap which needs rectifying. As described in Chapter 1, the approach is basing our clinical practice on the

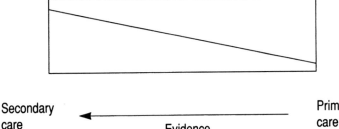

Secondary care Primary care

Evidence

Fig 2.3 Availability of evidence

best current evidence available. It makes our knowledge gaps explicit.

It is legitimate to start with what others have already done, beginning with overviews and practice guidelines rather than searching and appraising original research papers yourself. For example, we have already indicated that the use of published clinical guidelines on the management of systolic hypertension in the elderly would help in deciding how to treat Mrs D (Box 2.1); similarly, guidelines on the management of back pain would help one to respond to Mr X's request for referral to a chiropractor.[16] However, it is important to establish that the guidelines you use are based on evidence, as discussed in Chapter 9. Alternatively, overviews, such as the Effective Health Care Bulletin, can be used to guide management of, say, glue ear in children.[3]

For many problems presented by patients there will be no available clinical guidelines or overviews and it is then necessary to look for primary research studies of, say, the management of insomnia in the elderly and the role of melatonin in particular.[7]

Conclusion

In this chapter we have discussed the importance of getting the question right and which one to answer first. This leads to successful accession of the information on which to base our practice. We have also stressed the value of working together in this process which saves time and makes the approach more interesting.

References

1 McWhinney IR. *A textbook of family medicine*. Oxford: Oxford University Press, 1989.
2 Beard K, Bulpit C, Mascie-Taylor H, *et al*. Management of elderly patients with sustained hypertension. *BMJ* 1992;**304**:412–16.
3 The treatment of persistent glue ear in children. In: *Effective health care bulletin*, vol 1 (4). University of Leeds, 1992.

4 Balint M. *The doctor, his patient, and the illness*. London: Pitman Medical, 1964.

5 Woof WR, Carter YIL. The grieving adult and the general practitioner: a literature review in two parts (part 2). *Br J Gen Pract* 1997;**47**:443–8.

6 Evidence Based Care Resource Group. Evidence-based care. 1. Setting priorities: how important is this problem? *Can Med Assoc* 1994;**150**:1249–54.

7 Kirkwood CK. Management of insomnia. *J Am Pharm Assoc* 1999;**39**:688–96.

8 Sackett DL, Richardson WS, Rosenberg W, Haynes RB. *Evidence-based medicine: how to practice and teach EBM*. New York: Churchill Livingstone, 1997.

9 Sullivan FM, MacNaughton RJ. Evidence in consultations: interpreted and individualised. *Lancet* 1996;**348**:941–3.

10 Sackett DL, Rosenberg WMC, Gray JAM, Richardson WS. Evidence based medicine: what it is and what it isn't. *BMJ* 1996;**312**:71–2.

11 Roberts SJ, Harris CM. Age, sex, and temporary resident originated prescribing units (ASTRO-PUs): new weightings for analysing prescribing of general practices in England. *BMJ* 1993;**307**:485–8.

12 Armstrong D, Reyburn H, Jones R. A study of general practitioners' reasons for changing their prescribing behaviour. *BMJ* 1996;**312**:949–52.

13 Pringle M, Churchill R. Randomised controlled trials in general practice. *BMJ* 1995;**311**:382–3.

14 Bradley F, Field J. Evidence-based medicine. *Lancet* 1995;**346**:838.

15 Gill PS, Dowell AC, Neal RD, Smith N, Heywood P, Wilson AE. Evidence based general practice (authors' reply). BMJ 1996;**313**:114–15.

16 Royal College of General Practitioners. *National low back pain clinical guidelines*. London: RCGP, 1996.

3: Tracking down the evidence

CHRIS DEL MAR

Introduction

With over two million new research articles added to the world's health care literature each year,[1] there is certainly no shortage of information available to help inform clinical decision-making. The real challenge facing consumers and health care professionals is to be able to access effectively the information required to address their specific decision-making needs in a timely and efficient manner, and then to be able to use the information appropriately.[2]

This chapter explores a variety of ways to track down different types of evidence in order to help inform decision-making in general practice. The task goes beyond simply examining different methods of electronic searching to a deeper consideration of why the information is required in the first place. It is also important to examine who can use the information and how it can be used most effectively.

The general practitioner as an information broker

Traditionally, models of general practice have portrayed doctors as a "fount of knowledge", using their information and knowledge base to both educate and plan appropriate management for their patients. However, the information explosion of the twentieth century has made it impossible for doctors (or indeed any other health professionals) to keep up to date with all the available information. Furthermore, there is an increasing and important *emphasis* on shared decision-making in health care, which involves both health professionals and patients having access to similar information that forms the basis of discussion and negotiation, in order to arrive at a decision.[3,4] As a result, the role of health professionals is increasingly becoming more like that of information brokers, having responsibility for tracking down the necessary evidence (and often helping patients to do so as well) and then having the skills to help patients understand and interpret the information. In such an environment our credibility as health professionals stems not so much from what we know but our skill and ability to know how to know and transmit this to others.

Sources of information

The task of acting as an information broker is made more complex by the wide range of sources which both health professionals and patients can draw upon to inform decision-making. These range from traditional media (such as books and journal articles) to more interactive media (such as educational videos, CD-ROMs and the Internet). Unfortunately, not all sources provide information of equal quality or relevance.[5] Furthermore, not all sources are equally accessible to both health professionals and their patients.

Having decided upon the question or concern about which information is required, there is a series of five steps to take.

(1) Decide which type of information needs to be tracked down.
(2) Decide on the information sources that need to be checked.
(3) Develop efficient information retrieval strategies to access information from those sources.
(4) Scrutinise the quality and usefulness of the information obtained.
(5) Help patients understand and interpret the information.

Let us consider each of these steps in detail.

Step 1: decide which type of information needs to be tracked down

This is largely determined by the question that is to be answered. For example, the type of information required to answer a question about a patient's prognosis is very different from that required for a question about the symptoms the patient is likely to experience as a result of a particular treatment programme. In each case, the challenge is to identify information that can best help address the question in a reliable and useful way. The most influential factor in the decision about the type of information that needs to be tracked down is the study design. There is a range of different study designs (Figure 3.1), from experimental to observational, each of which has strengths and weaknesses depending on the question being asked.

Mrs C (Box 3.1) is a patient who poses questions for her GP that illustrate the requirement for different types of information.

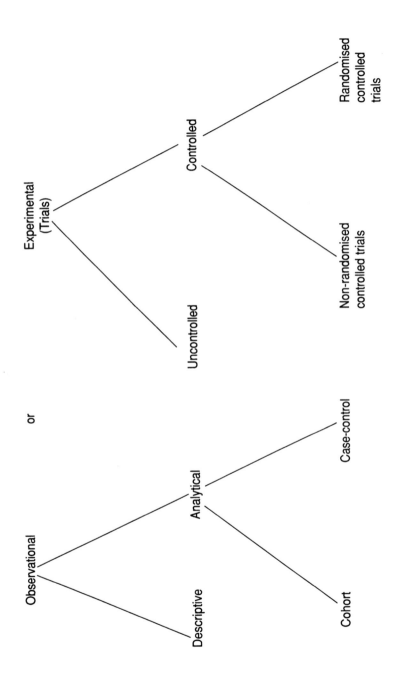

Fig 3.1 Types of studies

Box 3.1   Case study 1

Mrs C is a 37-year-old mother of two young children. She has been seeing her GP over the past two months with crippling joint pain in both hands. She has a family history of rheumatoid arthritis. Physical examination reveals a number of mildly swollen metacarpo-phalangeal joints in both hands. Her ESR (erythrocyte sedimentation rate) is 50 and rheumatoid factor is negative. She consults you asking three questions:

(1) What is the likelihood that she has rheumatoid arthritis with a negative rheumatoid factor?
(2) What type of functional limitations do people usually experience with rheumatoid arthritis?
(3) She has heard that aspirin can be effective in relieving symptoms and wants to know if it is more effective than the other non-steroida anti-inflammatory agents that are available.

Answering these questions requires tracking down different types of evidence in each case. For example, in collecting information that may help answer the question of what functional limitations are experienced by people with rheumatoid arthritis, good qualitative studies or prospective surveys using disability assessment instruments are both likely to be useful. However, neither of these types of evidence will give us much help in answering the question about diagnosis or treatment. For these questions we will be looking for the results of experiments, and, ideally, ones with control groups where patients have been randomised to receive either the intervention in question or the alternative we are interested in comparing it against.

Step 2: decide on the information sources that need to be checked

There are a large number of potential information sources to consider. Firstly, health professionals have their own personal knowledge base to draw on. In many cases, this knowledge base has developed as a result of undergraduate training and then been further developed as a result of postgraduate training and ongoing medical education. In the case of specialist medical practitioners, their knowledge base is often in a relatively narrow area but maintained by regular reading and attendance at scientific meetings. The danger with relying solely on the information base "possessed" by health professionals is that no matter how diligent we are in trying to keep up to date, we are rarely likely to have done so in a sufficiently comprehensive, systematic and rigorous manner. As a result, our knowledge base may be patchy or, at times, downright incorrect.[2] This may apply equally to specialists practising within a narrow field and general practitioners.

The second option is to consult with colleagues. This is the time-honoured method[2] and it has many advantages. Not only is it quick and convenient and achieves consistency with any other doctors also caring for the patient, it is relevant to local conditions and unlikely to lead to choices that are ludicrously unconventional. However, in common with textbooks (see below), the obvious drawback is that the information may be biased, out of date or simply derived only from past ritual and convention ("... this is what we always do...") that is not based on evidence. Moreover, when general practitioners consult specialist colleagues they may be given answers that have only limited application to primary care populations.

One excellent suggestion for getting the best evidence by consulting colleagues is to ask not just "What is the best treatment for...?" but also "... and what is the evidence for that?", for example, to enable an estimate of the level of evidence. Asking for the references and making sure that they are chased up adds another layer of stringency.

A third option is to draw on traditional media such as textbooks and journal articles. Unfortunately, these are frequently out of date by the time they are published, due to a considerable lag time from when evidence for some managements appears to the time the appropriate recommendations appear in textbooks.[6] Furthermore, there is evidence to show that many textbooks do not compile the primary research used to inform recommendations in a systematic manner. Nevertheless, there are some textbooks which are evidence-based.[7,8] Evidence-based texts will become more popular as an increasingly discriminating body of general practitioners demand more evidence for the advice offered in textbooks.

Journal articles do provide useful information, providing that one keeps in mind the variable quality of what is published and the fact that much completed research is never published. There is evidence of a systematic bias in some instances towards certain types of research being less likely to be published (for example, when the results are negative or equivocal compared with if the results are positive). The problem with relying on original journal articles is that there may be multiple articles that are relevant but widely scattered across different journals. It may therefore be extremely difficult to track down all the required articles.[1]

Review articles, which summarise and synthesise original research, offer a sensible way of helping both health professionals and patients keep up to date with the world's literature in a manageable way. However, in the past, many review articles have not been prepared in a systematic and rigorous manner and have therefore resulted in similar problems to those referred to with textbooks.[1] Fortunately, in recent years there has been a move towards encouraging a more systematic approach to reviewing original research. Organisations like the Cochrane Collaboration, which aims to prepare, maintain and promote the accessibility of systematic reviews on the benefits and risks of health care interventions, have been instrumental in this process.[8]

There are other ways in which original research can be summarised into forms that make the information more digestible to busy practitioners and their patients. For example, clinical practice guidelines are being prepared by many groups throughout the world for a range of different health care problems. Guidelines are considered in more detail in Chapter 9. For the purpose of this chapter, they provide one way in which relevant information is summarised and made more accessible. Many guidelines contain information written for both health professionals and patients.

A good health care librarian can be enormously helpful in assisting to track down textbooks, journal articles or guidelines. There are a number of electronic databases available which catalogue these different types of information. For example, MEDLINE is probably the most widely used electronic database of medical and health care journals, cataloguing about 3400 of the world's journals in this field (out of a total of 12 000–15 000). For practical purposes, it is the best starting point to identify health care information in general. Appendix 1 of this book gives details on how to search MEDLINE; only a small amount of training is required to become proficient in its use.

There are other electronic databases relevant to health care which cover different topic areas (see Appendices 1 and 2); for example, PSYCLIT is a database of journals in the field of psychology and mental health; CINAHL is a database of allied health and nursing journals. The *Cochrane Library*, produced by the Cochrane Collaboration, covers all of health care but only for a particular type of question: the effects of interventions. It would be a good starting point to search for information about the effectiveness of different treatment options for Mrs C (Box 3.1); however, it would not be a good place to search for information about the questions relating to diagnosis, qualitative experiences or incidence and extent of functional disability.

The *Cochrane Library* contains four separate databases:

(1) The Cochrane Database of Systematic Reviews, which consists of systematically compiled reviews of the effects of health care interventions.
(2) The Database of Abstracts of Reviews of Effectiveness, which consists of systematically compiled reviews of the effects of health care interventions published anywhere else in the world other than by the Cochrane Collaboration.
(3) The Cochrane Controlled Trials Register, which includes citations of controlled trials identified anywhere in the world's literature.
(4) The Cochrane Review Methodology Database, which is a bibliography of methodological papers relating to systematic reviews.[9]

"Instant" sources of evidence have become important. These attempt to sift material out of the medical literature that is both of adequate quality and clinical relevance – a tiny proportion of what is published. Research is collected by epidemiologists expert in the quality of published research, and screened by clinical "spotters" who decide on the clinical relevance. This is undertaken by electronic clubs such as *Bandolier* – http://www.jr2.ox.ac.uk/bandolier/index.html – and more formally by journals such as the *ACP* (*American College of Physicians*) *Journal Club* (a component of *Annals of Internal Medicine*) and combinations of journals such as *Best Evidence* (*ACP Journal Club* together with *Evidence-Based Medicine*), http://www.acponline.org/journals/acpjc/jcmenu.htm and Best Ev=http://hiru.mcmaster.ca/acpjc/acpod.htm]) which aims to select scientifically rigorous and clinically important information from a number of health care journals and present short abstracts and commentaries on these. The type of information covered is broader than the Cochrane Library and includes information about incidence, prognosis, risk and economic analysis, as well as information about studies of the effectiveness of health care interventions (also see Appendices 1 and 2).

Another innovation in this area comes in the form of something halfway between a journal and book called *Clinical Evidence*[10] – www.clinicalevidence.org – a sort of compendium of the best available evidence. It has even briefer summaries of the evidence for managing clinical problems. It looks like, and can be used as, a short half-life textbook. However, its contents deliver the information in an evidence-based way; that is, with a description of where the evidence comes from, and how strong it is. Moreover the information it contains is stored in a database to aid its review and update every 6 months. Buying a copy supplies you with a year's subscription; an updated version arrives 6 months hence.

The Internet represents the most widely used source of information that is increasingly available to almost anyone in our society. The Internet is able to facilitate access to large amounts of information that can be stored anywhere in the world. Increasingly, journals, textbooks and guidelines, previously available only in hard copy, are available on line. In addition, there are huge amounts of health care information written specifically for distribution on the Internet. Such information can vary from news announcements to educational information produced by health care organisations. Some of the information is targeted specifically at patients whilst other information may be directed towards both health professionals and patients. The task of searching for relevant information on the Internet is greatly aided by the existence of some very sophisticated "search engines" that allow inexperienced users to readily hone down on the information they require. There are also some useful guides to evidence-based information resources available on the Internet[11,12] (see also Appendix 2).

Whether or not we acquire the skills to access such information, we can be sure that some of our patients will do so very rapidly. The experience of patients coming in equipped with print-outs from Web sites is becoming increasingly familiar. Patients may often have managed to track down more recent or better information than their treating general practitioner is aware of (Box 3.2). Of course, the ability of the patient to access information sources such as the Internet represents an opportunity for general practitioners to share decision-making with the patient, and this is likely to increase the patient's sense of autonomy and ability to take increasing responsibility for his or her own health. There are several additional sources of health care information which have not been considered in detail here. These include the lay press, audiotapes, videos and interactive CD-ROMs. In most instances these sources contain information primarily oriented towards patients, although frequently they are also seen and used by health professionals. Unfortunately, there are usually no databases which catalogue such information so accessing it is more "hit or miss". In addition, the quality of the information can be much more variable than that from those sources which have been subjected to more formal peer review mechanisms.

Box 3.2   Case study 2

A woman came in with her 5-year-old son. The boy ran over to the box of toys and started playing happily. Mum placed a set of X-rays on the desk.

"While we were abroad on holiday, he fell and started limping," she said. "At the hospital over there they did these X-rays and said he has Perthes disease."

"I am so worried," she added. "I have looked at the Web page of a support group of Perthes disease and downloaded some stuff.... This picture of the splint really worried me!"

The boy was now fully recovered from his limp. The management therefore centred on dealing with interpreting the information his mother had obtained.

A word of warning. Many of the information sources described here (and particularly the Internet) can be extremely seductive. Before embarking on using them we should know what it is we are searching for, otherwise we run the risk of wasting a substantial amount of time and effort. It is a bit like flicking through a new journal to see if there is anything of interest. Even if we lay eyes on an interesting article, we must remember it needs to be interpreted in the context of other relevant articles in the area (to which we probably do not have ready access). Traditionally, most health professionals have regularly read one or two journals in their area. Because this is unlikely to be sufficient to cover all the necessary information to inform clinical decision-making, it is a far more efficient use of time to concentrate on searching for information which addresses only the specific clinical questions that we have.

Step 3: develop efficient information retrieval strategies to access information from those sources

The challenge with information retrieval is to avoid having to wade through large amounts of unnecessary information to find the few useful pieces that we need. Little time in this chapter will be spent discussing information retrieval strategies as these can be readily learnt using a few simple techniques. Table 3.1 summarises some useful starting-off points for different types of search and the sort of performance we can expect. Appendix 1 of this book contains practical adaptations of these "methodological filters", which reduce the time taken for them to run, and provides more detailed guidance on how to search the MEDLINE database. Often it may be helpful to seek additional expert assistance from a librarian.

Table 3.1   How good are search strategies at detecting "sound" articles?[13]

Type of study	Search strategy	Sensitivity	Specificity
Aetiology – the cause of the disease is of principle interest	EXP COHORT STUDIES or EXP RISK or ODDS(tw) and RATIO: (tw) or RELATIVE(tw) and RISK(tw) or CASE(tw) and CONTROL(tw)	0·82	0·70
Prognosis – the natural course of the disease is of principle interest	INCIDENCE or EXP MORTALITY or FOLLOW-UP STUDIES or MORTALITY(sh) or PROGNOS:(tw) or PREDICT:(tw) or COURSE:(tw)	0·92	0·73
Diagnosis – principle interest is in diagnostic tests	EXP SENSITIVITY AND SPECIFICITY or DIAGNOS &(px) or DIAGNOSTIC USE (sh) or SENSITIVITY (tw) or SPECIFICITY (tw)	0·92	0·73
Treatment/prevention – therapy, prevention, or rehabilitation is of principle interest	RANDOMISED CONTROLLED TRIAL(pt) or DRUG THERAPY(tw) or THERAPEUTIC USE (sh) or RANDOM:(tw)	0·99	0·74

(tw) = text word; (sh) = subject heading; &(px) = subheading before exploding the term; : = truncation of term, (pt) = publication type.
Note: These strategies apply specifically to MEDLINE, although the precise terms used can vary depending on the language of the search engine used. They are now automatically incorporated into the Web-based search facility of the National Library of Medicine (NLM) in Washington — {HYPERLINK http://www.ncbi.nlm.nih.gov/PubMed/}—
through a site called "Clinical Queries" –
{HYPERLINK http://www.ncbi.nlm.nih.gov:80/entrez/query/static/clinical.html }—
that has search engines within it that, for example, can search the "prognosis" question by simply pressing a button on the screen. Moreover it allows the search to be specific (return mostly useful material with little irrelevancies) or sensitive (miss little at the cost of returning much that is irrelevant). (see Appendix 2)
Similar strategies exist for other electronic databases and should be discussed with a librarian.

Step 4: scrutinise the quality and usefulness of the information obtained

Once we have found the information required, it is important to scrutinise its quality, keeping in mind its location in a relevant hierarchy of evidence. Although the formal skills required for this process (known as critical appraisal) will be considered in detail in Chapter 4, there are a number of simple checks that can be made on information to assess its likely quality and relevance. For example, we should always check the date when the information was prepared. If the only information is from many years ago, is it likely to be relevant still? Who prepared the information? Was it the work of a reputable organisation or individual, or is it from a less well-known source? This is particularly important in assessing information available on the Internet. If there are several trials suggesting the same answer, that is reassuring. Indeed, it is often reassuring to have information from several different sources (for example, case-control studies and randomised controlled trials, or the opinion of one's friendly specialist together with that of a meta-analysis) that establish the same direction and order of effect.

It is possible to conceptualise a hierarchy of evidence for different types of clinical question. The most frequently referred to hierarchy is for assessing information about risks and benefits associated with interventions; it reflects judgements about the value of different types of study design in minimising bias and is often used when preparing clinical practice guidelines in order to give readers some idea of the "grade of evidence". An example is given in Box 3.3.

The use of alternate hierarchies may be preferable for assessing the strength of evidence pertaining to other kinds of questions. For example, Table 3.3 shows how the hierarchy of study design can vary depending on the type of question asked, thus demonstrating that the most desirable study design for one type of question is not always the most appropriate for another question type (for example, while in Table 3.2 a cohort study is considered to be relatively "low level" evidence in the assessment of health care interventions, it would be considered highly desirable, or "high level" evidence for a prognosis question in Figure 3.2).

Step 5: help patients understand and interpret the information

This final step is probably the most crucial test of a health professional's ability to act as an information broker. Ideally, this ought to be a shared process, involving the health professional and the patient jointly discussing the evidence while taking into account the patient's preferences and/or values in order to arrive at a negotiated decision.[3,4] In some instances, patients may prefer less active involvement in the decision-making process, but still expect and appreciate thorough explanation of the doctor's

Box 3.3

Australian NHMRC designation of levels of evidence

I   evidence obtained from a systematic review of all relevant randomised controlled trials

II   evidence obtained from at least one properly designed randomised controlled trial

III-1 evidence obtained from well designed pseudo-randomised controlled trials (alternate allocation or some other method)

III-2 evidence obtained from comparative studies with concurrent controls and allocation not randomised (cohort studies), case-control studies, or interrupted time series with a control group

III-3 evidence obtained from comparative studies with historical control, two or more single-arm studies, or interrupted time series without a parallel control group

IV   evidence obtained from case series, either post-test or pre-test and post-test.

These levels of evidence ratings have been adapted from US Preventive Services Task Force (1989), Guide to clinical preventive services: an assessment of the effectiveness of 169 interventions (ed. M Fisher), Williams and Williams, Baltimore, Appendix A, p. 388.

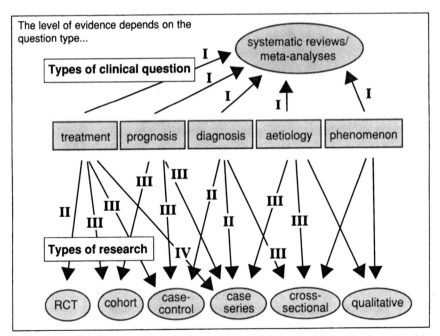

Figure 3.2 Levels of evidence[14] (Thanks to Paul Glasziou for help in this figure.)

recommendations.[3,4] With the growth in evidence-based patient information material and resources, it ought to be possible for all patients to have access to reliable supporting information about the decision(s) that need to be made.[5] It is beyond the scope of this chapter to address this issue; however, the interpretation and application of information by general practitioners in conjunction with their patients forms the basis of Chapter 5.

A practical example

Case study 3 (Box 3.4) represents a clinical problem that illustrates how the five steps referred to in this chapter can be applied in practice.

Keeping up to date and tracking down evidence

Most of this chapter has focused on tracking down evidence in response to specific clinical questions. This approach should be useful for most GPs and patients as, for many, it is the major reason that they access health care literature. The traditional concept of reading a selected list of journals as part of a continuing education strategy in order to keep up to date is becoming increasingly inappropriate as the amount of information available increases exponentially and becomes even more widely distributed amongst the growing number of health care journals.

Unless you have plenty of time to browse through medical journals, focus on reading to solve specific areas of clinical uncertainty or need. If you want to make sure you keep abreast of new developments relevant to general practice, and only want to read one or two journals, try reading a journal like *Evidence-based Medicine* or the *ACP Journal Club*, both of which summarise key articles from other journals. Even with these journals, you need to be very discriminating – ruthless even – in what you read. Check the title, and if it seems interesting and/or relevant to your practice, go on and read the abstract to see if you are still interested. If so, it may be worthwhile to go back and get the original article and read it in detail. Alternatively, you may find that there is sufficient information for your purposes in the published abstract and the commentary provided on the article.

Many GPs find the idea of keeping up to date on their own rather daunting. It may be helpful to talk to others about their discoveries, and to hear about the discoveries of others in turn. One very good method of undertaking this is to form a journal club. Here, a group of similar-minded doctors meet regularly and discuss their readings from the journals and share their discoveries. In particular, it may be aided by nominating how any particular article will be useful in clinical practice. "From now on, I will..." is the sort of practice-changing intention that will indicate that the process is worthwhile. Strategies to promote the implementation of evidence in primary care, and the assessment of the effectiveness of its implementation are discussed further in Part 2 of this book.

Box 3.4   Case study 3

Mr S was a 47-year-old who presented to his GP for an insurance medical examination. He had no previous relevant medical history. One of the requirements was for a urine test. This was tested by the practice nurse and returned "blood – moderate". The abnormality was confirmed with a urine microscopy and culture. The culture was negative but morphologically normal red cells in a concentration of 30 per high power field were present. Examination of Mr S was normal, in particular his blood pressure and abdomen. Should he be investigated further?

His GP recalled from his medical education the common causes of microscopic haematuria (general causes such as anticoagulation, glomerular causes such as IgA glomerulonephritis and finally lesions of the transition cell epithelium, including transitional cell carcinoma). Some of these are clearly life threatening. Should they be excluded?

He called up two of his friendly urologists in turn. One said, "Yes, well I believe all cases of microscopic haematuria should be investigated to determine the source of the bleeding; I have seen nasty cancers missed by delay where I may have been able to effect a cure." The other said "Only 30 cells per high power field? Well the chances of anything nasty are very small – no, I can't tell exactly how small – and we don't want to go investigating unnecessarily, do we?"

A quick look at the Cochrane Database of Systematic Reviews revealed no information there on this subject. (On the Cochrane Controlled Trials Register there were 18 hits for "Haematuria" and 40 for "Hematuria", and although a few dealt with diagnosis – ultrasound vs intravenous urography, for example – there were none that helped with the prognosis.)

The GP decided to undertake a search. The searching equipment at the practice consisted of a computer with a modem, linked to the local hospital library, accessing MEDLINE on a CD. The library had supplied software to enable outside subscribers to search the CD drive from the outside.

The search strategy in Table 3.1 under "Prognosis – the natural course of the disease is of principle interest" was used as the relevant one for this situation. The search terms were adapted for the particular search engine of the software (called WIN-SPIRS or Mac-SPIRS, Silver Platter Information Retrieval System for Windows or Macintosh):

i.e. "INCIDENCE OR EXP MORTALITY OR FOLLOW UP STUDIES OR
MORTALITY(sh) OR PROGNOS:(tw) OR PREDICT:(tw) OR COURSE:(tw)"

was converted into the following search, with the added result of urinalysis:

(INCIDENCE OR EXPLODE (MORTALITY OR (FOLLOW UP STUDIES) OR
MORTALITY OR PROGNOS: OR PREDICT: OR COURSE)) AND
(HEMATURIA OR HAEMATURIA)

This relatively unsophisticated search revealed 223 hits after a search that took about 10 minutes. The doctor was inclined simply to look through the titles of all these. Rather than look at them "live", the connection with the library was closed down after downloading all the titles. (Costs for this practice were based not on the number of abstracts downloaded but on the time linked to the library's computer). The references were then loaded into a software program that managed the doctor's references. Opening this allowed the references to be examined at leisure. About half could be removed just from inspection of the titles (many were about people with follow up after malignancy, people with bleeding disorders and with other serious conditions such as AIDS that were not relevant to Mr S). The doctor browsed through the 100 or so left. This took the best part of an evening. Among these were two that were extremely relevant: a screening for haematuria program in the USA which described the outcomes compared to controls from outside the programme and a study of the outcomes of air force men, similarly screened for haematuria, who were investigated. All was very reassuring for the doctor and Mr S when they discussed the results along with the options. Together they elected to postpone further investigations and adopt a wait-and-see management approach, in particular, asking Mr S to return should he develop any symptoms.

The effort may have saved considerable expense and anxiety for the patient.
Another way of undertaking this search would be to use the free search site of the Web-based MEDLINE service of the US National Library of Medicine – http://www.ncbi.nlm.nih.gov/PubMed/ – particularly the site within it called "Clinical Queries" – http://www.ncbi.nlm.nih.gov:80/entrez/query/static/clinical.html (see Table 3.1).

Whatever personal strategy is used to try to keep abreast of developments, the effort of remembering and retrieving the information obtained will always be made easier by keeping a personal record. As with so many other aspects of office life, this challenge has been made immeasurably easier by the use of software packages specifically designed for keeping bibliographies.[2]

Conclusion

As the role of general practitioners changes from being the "fount of all knowledge" to an "information broker", the skills of tracking down the evidence will become as core as the skills of history taking and physical examination. It is likely that new systems and technologies will continue to be developed to assist health care professionals and patients access information. Despite these advances, the challenge of ensuring that the information obtained is of high quality and appropriately applied will remain for the foreseeable future.

References

1 Mulrow CD. Rationale for systematic reviews. In: Chalmers I, Altman DG, eds. *Systematic reviews*. London: BMJ Publishing Group, 1995.
2 Smith R. What clinical information do doctors need? *BMJ* 1996;**313**:1062–8.
3 Charles C, Gafni A, Whelan T. Shared decision-making in the medical encounter: what does it mean (or it takes at least two to tango). *Soc Sci Med* 1997;**44**:681–92.
4 Sutherland HJ, Llewellyn-Thomas HA, Lockwood GA, *et al.* Cancer patients: their desire for information and participation in treatment decisions. *J Roy Soc Med* 1989;**82**:260.
5 Entwistle VA, Sheldon TA, Sowden AJ, Watt IS. Supporting consumer involvement in decision-making: what constitutes quality in consumer health information? *Int J Quality Health Care* 1996;**8**:425–37.
6 Antman EM, Lau J, Kupelnick B, *et al.* A comparison of the results of meta-analyses of randomised control trials and recommendations of clinical experts. Treatments for myocardial infarction. *JAMA* 1992;**268**:240–8.
7 Panzer RJ, Black ER, Griner PF, eds. *Diagnostic strategies for common medical problems*. Philadelphia, PA: American College of Physicians Press, 1991.
8 Goroll A, Mulley AG. *Primary care medicine: office evaluation and management of the adult patient*. Philadelphia, PA: Lippincott, 1995.

9 Bero L, Drummond R. The Cochrane Collaboration. Preparing, maintaining, and disseminating systematic reviews of the effects of health care. *JAMA* 1995;**274**:1935–8.

10 Godlee F. *Clinical evidence. A compendium of the best available evidence for effective health care.* London: BMJ Publications, 2000.

11 Zack M. Index of EBM resources on the WWW. www.ohsu.edu/biccc-informatics/ebm/index.html.

12 Medical Matrix. www.medmatrix.org/index.asp.

13 Haynes RB. Developing optimal search strategies for detecting clinically sound studies in MEDLINE. *J Am Med Informatics Assoc* 1994;**1**:447–58.

14 Commonwealth of Australia. *How to use the evidence: assessment and application of scientific evidence.* Canberra: Biotext, 2000. www.health.gov.au/nhmrc/publicat/synopses/cp65syn.htm.

4: Critical appraisal

TIM LANCASTER AND MICHAEL WEINGARTEN

Introduction

Critical appraisal is the ability to read original research, to make a judgement on its scientific value, and to consider how its results can be applied in practice. There are two main issues in critical appraisal: (1) to determine whether the study has been properly conducted and the results can therefore be trusted; (2) to decide whether the results can be used in practice.

Before deciding to apply the results of a published study we need to know how far we can rely on them. Results may be relied upon inasmuch as the measurements were made properly and reproducibly. Are the results valid? Validity depends on the measures taken to reduce sources of bias, for example, whether there was random allocation of treatment in studies of the effectiveness of therapy. Many clinicians lack confidence in assessing reliability and validity because they perceive themselves to have a poor knowledge of issues in study design. In practice, they can rapidly learn to make accurate judgements about this issue by following a few simple principles. This task has been made much easier by the development and testing of non-technical guidelines for assessing the quality of evidence. A variety are available and they have tended to evolve into increasingly simple forms. The journal series entitled "Users' guides to the medical literature", which appeared in the *Journal of the American Medical Association*, is a good starting point. This series includes articles on how to appraise studies in core topics of clinical practice such as therapy, diagnosis, prognosis and aetiology.[1-8] In addition, there are guides to assessing the quality of different forms of research synthesis, including reviews, decision analysis, guidelines and audit.[9-16] Although the questions asked of each study vary depending on the topic of the paper, the series suggests a core series of questions to ask of any paper: What were the results? Are the results of the study valid? Will the results help me in caring for my patients?

This approach has been further refined in a recent textbook which includes pocket-card outlines.[17] More recently still, authors who had been involved in developing both these resources suggested that the "bare bones" of this approach could be reduced to two or three questions for each type of study (Table 4.1).[18]

Table 4.1   Bare bones users' guides for appraisal of the validity of medical studies

Purpose of study	Guides		
Therapy	Concealed random allocation of patients to comparison groups	Outcome measure of known or probable clinical importance	Few lost to follow-up compared with number of bad outcomes
Diagnosis	Patients to whom you would want to apply the test in practice	Objective or reproducible diagnostic standard, applied to all participants	Blinded assessment of test and diagnostic standards
Prognosis	Inception cohort, early in the course of the disorder and initially free of the outcome of interest	Objective or reproducible assessment of clinically important outcomes	Few lost to follow-up compared with number of bad outcomes
Aetiology	Clearly identified comparison group or those at risk for, or having, the outcome of interest	Blinding of observers of outcome to exposure; blinding of observers of exposure to outcome	
Reviews	Explicit criteria for selecting articles and rating validity	Comprehensive search for all relevant articles	

Applying criteria such as these, learners rapidly acquire confidence in detecting bias which may threaten the validity of reported research. Indeed, one problem faced by teachers of critical appraisal is to rein these skills in once learnt: overenthusiastic criticism of study methodology may end up in nihilism. It is important to be able to detect fatal flaws so that precious reading time is not spent on papers that have nothing to offer. But it is also important to appreciate that evidence can be helpful without being perfect.

Perhaps the best way to avoid getting bogged down in criticism of study methods is to focus on the second part of critical appraisal – deciding what the results are and how far they are applicable in practice. A distinctive contribution of evidence-based medicine has been to focus on the ways research evidence is presented, for example, in the use of likelihood ratios for assessing the value of diagnostic tests, and numbers needed to treat (NNT) as a method of expressing the magnitude of treatment effects.[19,20]

Here, in our first example, we show how we used critical appraisal of the evidence in a recent clinical problem in primary care.

Example 1

A 67-year-old man (Mr J) attended the surgery in a distressed state. His brother, who lived in another town, had died suddenly of a heart attack the week before, aged 56. In addition to his bereavement, Mr J was very anxious about his own future risk of cardiovascular disease. He wanted to know what the implications were for him, and what he could do to reduce his risk. Specifically, he wondered whether he should be taking a cholesterol-lowering drug. His records showed that he had suffered an inferior myocardial infarction at the age of 64. He had given up smoking at the time of his myocardial infarction and was not overweight. He had no current symptoms of angina, blood pressure was 132/84, and two successive cholesterol measurements had been greater than 8.0 mmol/l despite attempting to follow a diet low in saturated fat. His body mass index was 29 kg/m^2 and he had repeatedly attempted to follow weight-reducing diets. There was no history of diabetes.

We suggested that he had repeat cholesterol and high density lipoprotein (HDL) cholesterol measurements and that he come back for a follow-up appointment. In the meantime we wrote to the brother's doctor for further details. He replied that the brother had died of acute coronary thrombosis. He had been overweight, took little exercise, was being treated for hypertension, and had had a series of cholesterol measurements, ranging from 7.7 mmol/l to 6.6 mmol/l after dietary advice. He did not smoke.

Follow-up lipid measurements on Mr J were total cholesterol of 7.9 mmol/l and HDL cholesterol of 1.2 mmol/l.

Aware of recent new research on treating elevated cholesterol levels, we decided to see how the evidence could help with this patient. Since he had a cholesterol level higher than the recommended level after dietary treatment, we were interested in whether, and by how much, drug treatment to lower cholesterol might reduce his risk of cardiovascular disease.

We located a study of cholesterol lowering in patients with elevated cholesterol and established cardiovascular disease, the 4S study, comparing . . . patients.[21]

What were the results?

We first examined the results of the study. Overall, after approximately five years, 11.5% of patients in the placebo group had died, compared to 8.2% in the simvastatin group. This meant that the relative risk of dying (the rate in the simvastatin group divided by the rate in the placebo group) was 70%. In other words, those treated with simvastatin had a reduction in the relative risk of dying of 30%. This sounded promising, but the relative risk is a difficult concept to use clinically. It does not take account of the individual patient's absolute risk of having the outcome of interest. A 30% reduction in risk might be very important clinically if the risk of developing the condition was common, but trivial if that risk was small.

Another way of considering the figures is to look at the absolute risk reduction (the risk in the placebo group minus the risk in the treatment group). This was 11.5 −8.2, or 3.3%. This still does not immediately make clinical sense, so we converted the absolute risk reduction to numbers needed to treat (NNT) (which is conveniently done by taking the reciprocal of the absolute risk reduction, or 1/0.033). This showed that we would have to treat 30 patients with simvastatin for 5 years to prevent one death. Similar calculations showed that the NNT for combined fatal and non-fatal coronary events was 15, and for coronary surgery/angioplasty was 17. The likelihood of adverse events did not differ between the treatment and placebo group (Table 4.2).

Table 4.2 Calculations that can be used to analyse the results of the Scandinavian Simvastatin Survival Study (4S)[21]

Measure	Definition	Calculations	
		Equation	Data
Relative Risk (RR)	The risk of an outcome (dying) if exposed to the intervention (treatment with simvastatin), as opposed to comparator (placebo)	S/P	8.2/11.5=70%
Absolute Risk Reduction (ARR)	The reduction in absolute risk of an outcome (dying) – depends on baseline risk	S−P	11.5−8.2=3.3%
Number Needed To Treat (NNT)	The number of patients that would need to be exposed to the intervention (treatment with simvastatin for 5 years) to prevent 1 outcome (death)	1/ARR	1/0.033=30

Were the results valid?

A rapid screen convinced us that the study was scientifically valid. The study was a double-blind randomised controlled trial, all the patients were followed up, and the analysis was performed according to the groups to which the patients were allocated (intention to treat). Finally, the study was designed to be large (powerful) enough to give reliable (statistically significant) answers about the effect of the treatment on total mortality as well as on different types of cardiovascular disease outcomes (fatal and non-fatal myocardial infarction, coronary surgery and angioplasty).

Were the results applicable?

The last step was to determine what types of patients were studied and how closely they resembled our patient. The subjects of the study included men and women aged 35–70 with a history of angina or myocardial infarction whose total cholesterol after dietary treatment was 5.3-8.0 mmol/l. Mr J would therefore have been eligible to enter the study, and we felt confident that the results could be applied to him.

We were able to explain to Mr J that cholesterol-lowering drugs for him and other patients like him had a measurable chance of helping him and that they were very unlikely to harm him. He was offered, and accepted, treatment.

Our second example is about choosing a test for a screening programme in the practice.

Example 2

Following the detection of a couple of cases of colorectal cancer in our practice, we thought we ought to be trying harder to diagnose this condition earlier. We were aware of the debate about the value of faecal occult blood screening, and that the issue was still undecided, but nonetheless we decided to go ahead, offering annual faecal blood testing to all our patients over the age of 50. The question was, which kit to use?

Once again we found an article[22] on which we could base our choice which compared several different test kits: 10 702 members of an American health care organisation, Kaiser Permanente, were offered the screening test over a one-year period. The stool samples were tested using three different kits, Hemoccult II, Hemoccult II Sensa and HemeSelect. The screened patients were followed up two years later for the development of neoplasms (colorectal cancer or a polyp greater than 1 cm in diameter) from the organisation's cancer registry project and from the local pathology departments.

We used the same series of critical questions to assess the results of the study.

What were the results?

The sensitivities (see also p. 69) of the tests in diagnosing colorectal cancer were reported to range from 37% to 79%, so some cases would be missed, and their specificities were from 87% to 98%, so we might expect there to be relatively few false-positives. We needed to know more than that; we wanted to know how far these false-positives and negatives would affect our work in practice. In other words, what would be the frequency of false alarms with the different tests and what would be the frequency of false reassurance? The performance of the tests in practice depends on the prevalence of colorectal cancer in the population being screened. For a very rare disease, even a test with a high specificity will produce a larger number of false-positive results than true positives. In this study they found cancer at a frequency of 4.3 per 1000 (0.43%). Table 4.3 shows how the three rates – sensitivity. specificity, and prevalence – are sufficient to provide the information we needed.

Table 4.3   Assessing diagnostic tests: sensitivity, specificity and predictive values

		Disease		
		Present	Absent	Total
Test	Positive	a	b	a+b
	Negative	c	d	c+d
	Total	a+c	b+d	

Definitions

Sensitivity: a/(a+c)   False-negative rate: c/(a+c)
Specificity: d/(b+d)   False-positive rate: b/(b+d)

Positive predictive value: a/(a+b)   False alarm rate: b/(a+b)
Negative predictive value: d/(c+d)   False reassurance rate: c/(c+d)

Using their data, the authors calculated figures for the positive predictive values, between 2.5% and 6.6%, meaning that in the vast majority of cases, with all three tests, a positive result would not mean that the patient had colorectal cancer. The false alarm rate (1 – positive predictive value) would be between 93.4% and 97.5%. Conversely, a negative result would sometimes provide false reassurance. The false reassurance rates (1 – negative predictive value) were extremely low – between 0.1% and 0.3%.

Hemoccult II had the lowest sensitivity, and Hemoccult II Sensa had the highest sensitivity but the lowest specificity. HemeSelect occupied an intermediate position for both sensitivity and specificity. The authors concluded that the best strategy for screening was to use HemeSelect or a combination using Hemoccult II Sensa and HemeSelect to confirm positive results. The combination approach gave the highest positive predictive value, of 9%.

Were the results valid?

The study compared the results of the three different test kits on the same stool specimens, avoiding any bias related to the patients being examined. However, since Hemoccult II Sensa is more likely to be influenced by diet because of its higher sensitivity to peroxidase activity, poor compliance with dietary restriction would increase the positivity rate with this test more than with the others. This is pointed out by the authors in their discussion.

The tests were developed and interpreted by trained technicians at the medical centre and at the producers' laboratories, with periodical checks to monitor quality. Unusable cards were discarded and excluded from the analysis. This may have led to an underestimate of true sensitivity, but reflects reality.

The results are given as percentages with 95% confidence intervals, so that we may assess the range within which the tests might be expected to perform in practice. For example, the positive predictive value for the combination of Hemoccult II Sensa and HemeSelect is 9% with a confidence interval of 5.8–13.6%.

Since assessing the performance of these tests is so dependent on the diagnosis of the disease when present, we must be convinced that the follow-up was sufficient to detect all cases which developed. The method of 2-year follow-up rather than colonoscopies for all is a realistic and valid way of doing this. Follow-up data were available for 96% of the patients screened, and for another 2% there was 1-year follow-up data available. So even if one carcinoma was missed, this would essentially make no difference to the results.

The rates of detection of polyps greater than 1? cm which might be premalignant were also reported, but since these polyps may not always start bleeding within two years, the method of follow-up was not a sufficiently reliable way of detecting all of them.

In summary, the results could be accepted as valid for our purposes, i.e. screening for established colorectal carcinoma.

Were the results applicable?

The population used in the study may not have been comparable to our own since it seemed, from reading the article, that they derived from those people who chose to avail themselves of a "personal health appraisal", comprising a questionnaire, a physical examination and laboratory tests. This setting might be significantly different from the unselected population of a general practitioner's list. Patients who use preventive health care programmes may be different in several relevant ways from the general population. On the other hand, this should make no difference to the results comparing the three test kits, only possibly to the compliance rate and to the prevalence of positive findings. So in this aspect, we concluded that we could reasonably apply the findings in our decision.

The combination of Hemoccult II Sensa and HemeSelect is not available commercially, making it unpracticable to apply the authors' recommendation. Furthermore, the strategy of confirming a positive result on one test by retesting with another test leaves us with nagging doubts when the second test does not confirm the positive finding. Perhaps the patient bled sporadically and really does have a tumour? So in a clinical setting, this strategy is problematic.

The test collection kits were supplied to the patients who had to apply consecutive stool specimens to three test cards, using paper collecting devices designed to allow the sampling of the stool before it made contact with the water in the toilet bowl. The completed cards were submitted to the medical centre within three days after starting to collect the specimens and developed within 48 hours by the laboratory. The best test, HemeSelect, was also the most likely to be influenced by faulty collection technique, such as poor compliance with dietary restrictions before testing, small sample size and uneven spreading of the sample on the card. There were many more unusable cards with this test than with the others. Also, the cost of HemeSelect was six to seven times as high as the other tests.

If we were considering a more restricted screening programme for higher risk patients only, such as those with first-degree relatives with colorectal cancer, the pre-test probability of disease would be as high, therefore the screening test would be more powerful. The most useful way of dealing with this issue is to derive a likelihood ratio for a positive result, which is the ratio of sensitivity: (1 − specificity) (see also p. 69), from the data and apply it to Fagan's nomogram (Figure 4.1).[23] This shows how the test will predict disease with greater certainty, the higher the pre-test probability. The authors did not calculate likelihood ratios for us so we would have to do this ourselves if we wanted to consider a more selective high risk population approach. Simple arithmetic provided us with a range of likelihood ratios for the three tests of 6–16, and if colorectal cancer is 10 times more common, say, in high-risk patients than in the general population, we see that the chances of illness in the presence of a positive test are in the region of 30%, whichever test is used.

Taking all these reservations into consideration, we concluded that in practice we preferred a higher sensitivity and not to risk false-negatives, so we chose to use Hemoccult II Sensa whose characteristics we now knew to be: sensitivity 79.4%; specificity 86.7%; false alarm rate 97.5%; false reassurance rate 0.1%.

Conclusion

In this chapter we have not set out to provide a guide to critically appraising a paper. There are now a number of such guides available and we suggest that readers consult one of the sources we have mentioned. Instead, we have set out to show how critical appraisal can be used to help in solving clinical problems. Busy family doctors may feel too much time is

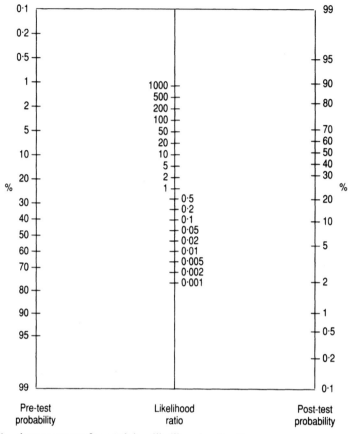

Fig 4.1 A nomogram for applying likelihood ratios.[23]

required to work through problems in the way we have described. We chose these problems deliberately because they are common and come up in our practice again and again. We anticipate the time taken over these problems will be repaid many times over as we apply the evidence to other patients and situations. As clinicians, we feel that, provided the topic is important to us and common, critically appraising the evidence in this way is an efficient method of keeping ourselves up to date.

References

1 Oxman AD, Sackett DL, Guyatt GH. Users' guides to the medical literature. I. How to get started. The Evidence-Based Medicine Working Group. *JAMA* 1993;**270**:2093–5.

2 Guyatt GH, Sackett DL, Cook DJ. Users' guides to the medical literature. II. How to use an article about therapy or prevention. A. Are the results of the study valid? The Evidence-Based Medicine Working Group. *JAMA* 1993;**270**:2598–601.

3 Guyatt GH, Sackett DL, Cook DJ. Users' guides to the medical literature. II. How to use an article about therapy or prevention. B. What were the results and will they help me in caring for my patients? The Evidence-Based Medicine Working Group. *JAMA* 1994;271:59–63.

4 Jaeschke R, Guyatt G, Sackett DL. Users' guides to the medical literature. III. How to use an article about a diagnostic test. A. Are the results of the study valid? The Evidence-Based Medicine Working Group. *JAMA* 1994;271:389–91.

5 Jaeschke R, Guyatt GH, Sackett DL. Users' guides to the medical literature. III. How to use an article about a diagnostic test. B. What are the results and will they help me in caring for my patients? The Evidence-Based Medicine Working Group. *JAMA* 1994;271:703–7.

6 Levine M, Walter S, Lee H, Haines T, Holbrook A, Moyer V. Users' guides to the medical literature. IV. How to use an article about harm. The Evidence-Based Medicine Working Group. *JAMA* 1994;271:1615–19.

7 Laupacis A, Wells G, Richardson WS, Tugwell P. Users' guides to the medical literature. V. How to use an article about prognosis. The Evidence-Based Medicine Working Group. *JAMA* 1994;272:234–7.

8 Richardson WS, Wilson MC, Guyatt GH, Cook DJ, Nishikawa J. Users' guides to the medical literature. XV. How to use an article about disease probability for differential diagnosis. Evidence-Based Medicine Working Group. *JAMA* 1999;281:1214–19.

9 Oxman AD, Cook DJ, Guyatt GH. Users' guides to the medical literature. VI. How to use an overview. The Evidence-Based Medicine Working Group. *JAMA* 1994;272:1367–71.

10 Richardson WS, Detsky AS. Users' guides to the medical literature. VII. How to use a clinical decision analysis. A. Are the results of the study valid? The Evidence-Based Medicine Working Group. *JAMA* 1995;273:1292–5.

11 Hayward RS, Wilson MC, Tunis SR, Bass EB, Guyatt G. Users' guides to the medical literature. VIII. How to use clinical practice guidelines. A. Are the recommendations valid? The Evidence-Based Medicine Working Group. *JAMA* 1995;274:570–4.

12 Guyatt GH, Sackett DL, Sinclair JC, Hayward R, Cook DJ, Cook RJ. Users' guides to the medical literature. IX. A method for grading health care recommendations. The Evidence-Based Medicine Working Group. *JAMA* 1995;274:1800–4.

13 Naylor CD, Guyatt GH. Users' guides to the medical literature. X. How to use an article reporting variations in the outcomes of health services. The Evidence-Based Medicine Working Group. *JAMA* 1996;275:554–8.

14 Naylor CD, Guyatt GH. Users' guides to the medical literature. XI. How to use an article about a clinical utilization review. The Evidence-Based Medicine Working Group. *JAMA* 1996;275:1435–9.

15 Drummond MF, Richardson WS, O'Brien BJ, Levine M, Heyland D. Users' guides to the medical literature. XIII. How to use an article on economic analysis of clinical practice. A. Are the results of the study valid? The Evidence-based Medicine Working Group. *JAMA* 1997;277:1552–7.

16 O'Brien BJ, Heyland D, Richardson WS, Levine M, Drummond MF. Users' guides to the medical literature. XIII. How to use an article on economic analysis of clinical practice. B. What are the results and will they help me in caring for my patients? Evidence-Based Medicine Working Group. *JAMA* 1977;277:1802–6.

17 Sackett DL, Richardson WS, Rosenberg W, Haynes RB. *Evidence-based medicine. How to practice and teach EBM*. London: Churchill Livingstone, 1997.

18 Haynes RB, Sackett DL, Muir Gray JA, Cook DL, Guyatt GH. Transferring evidence from research into practice: 2. Getting the evidence straight. *Evidence-based Med* 1997;**1**:4–6.

19 Laupacis A, Sackett DL, Roberts RS. An assessment of clinically useful measures of the consequences of treatment. *N J Engl Med* 1988;**318**:1728–33.

20 Chatelier G, Zapletal E, Lemaitre D, Menard J, Degoulet P. Number needed to treat: a clinically useful nomogram in its proper context. *BMJ* 1996;**312**:426–9.

21 Scandinavian Simvastatin Survival Study Group. Randomised trial of cholesterol lowering in 4444 patients with coronary heart disease: the Scandinavian Simvastatin Survival Study (4S). *Lancet* 1994;**344**:1383–9.

22 Allison JE, Tekawa IS, Ransom LJ, Adrain AL. A comparison of fecal occult-blood tests for colorectal-cancer screening. *N Engl J Med* 1996;**334**:155–9.

23 Fagan TJ. Nomogram for Bayes' theorem. *N Engl J Med* 1975;**293**:257.

5: Applying the evidence with patients

TRISHA GREENHALGH AND GAVIN YOUNG

General practice is *par excellence* the place where guilt accumulates in direct proportion to the growing stack of unopened journals.[1] The skill of the generalist has always lain in choosing what to ignore, and the challenge of the busy general practitioner is to identify and interpret *relevant* evidence for guiding decision-making in the surgery and at the bedside. This chapter will demonstrate, using case histories, how we tried to do this in four real-life situations.

General practitioners have a long tradition of analysing the psychosocial aspects of their encounters with patients,[2,3] and as Sullivan and MacNaughton have shown, accessing and appraising scientific evidence is a crucial but limited aspect of the primary care consultation (Figure 5.1).[4] Nevertheless, the general practitioner of the 21st century will depend increasingly on his or her ability to access relevant information (as described in Chapter 3), and to convert selected snippets of bald data, such as a number-needed-to-treat for a particular intervention, into patient-orientated clinical wisdom ("*this* patient should be advised to take *this* treatment at *this* point in time").[1]

The evidence-based approach to patient care advocated by Sackett and colleagues[5] presented a paradigm shift for medical science in the early 1990s. It was no longer the doctor's authority, but the nature and strength of the evidence that should justify (or proscribe) a particular clinical decision.[6] But as the pioneers of the evidence-based approach quickly discovered, even when valid, consistent and unambiguous evidence exists for a specific manoeuvre in a given set of clinical circumstances (and that is a rare enough situation), the "ideal" course of action is seldom a foregone conclusion.[7]

For one thing, the ideal option may be unaffordable within available resources. For another, practical barriers to implementation (such as time constraints on the clinician, lack of relevant skills or restricted availability of laboratory tests) may exist.[8] In many cases, the "textbook" management

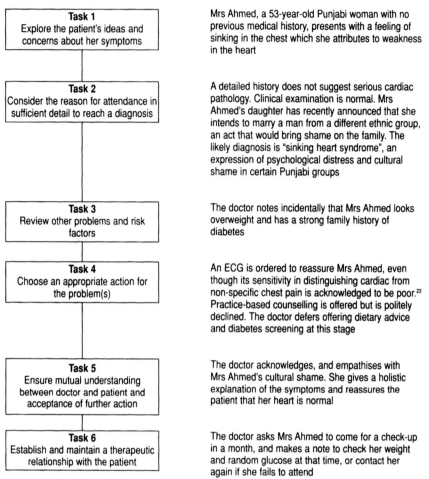

Task 1 Explore the patient's ideas and concerns about her symptoms	Mrs Ahmed, a 53-year-old Punjabi woman with no previous medical history, presents with a feeling of sinking in the chest which she attributes to weakness in the heart
Task 2 Consider the reason for attendance in sufficient detail to reach a diagnosis	A detailed history does not suggest serious cardiac pathology. Clinical examination is normal. Mrs Ahmed's daughter has recently announced that she intends to marry a man from a different ethnic group, an act that would bring shame on the family. The likely diagnosis is "sinking heart syndrome", an expression of psychological distress and cultural shame in certain Punjabi groups
Task 3 Review other problems and risk factors	The doctor notes incidentally that Mrs Ahmed looks overweight and has a strong family history of diabetes
Task 4 Choose an appropriate action for the problem(s)	An ECG is ordered to reassure Mrs Ahmed, even though its sensitivity in distinguishing cardiac from non-specific chest pain is acknowledged to be poor.[23] Practice-based counselling is offered but is politely declined. The doctor defers offering dietary advice and diabetes screening at this stage
Task 5 Ensure mutual understanding between doctor and patient and acceptance of further action	The doctor acknowledges, and empathises with Mrs Ahmed's cultural shame. She gives a holistic explanation of the symptoms and reassures the patient that her heart is normal
Task 6 Establish and maintain a therapeutic relationship with the patient	The doctor asks Mrs Ahmed to come for a check-up in a month, and makes a note to check her weight and random glucose at that time, or contact her again if she fails to attend

Fig 5.1 Task-orientated analysis of the general practice consultation.[2,4]

option will be modified by particular patient circumstances such as co-morbidity or additional risk factors. Furthermore, even when both the patient and the health professional have read and fully understood the same evidence, they may not both agree, for example, that taking a tablet every morning for blood pressure control is worth the effort, that continuous fetal heart monitoring is a reassurance rather than an intrusion during labour or that an upper gastrointestinal endoscopy is a minor diagnostic procedure. In other words, the patient and the health professional may assign different *utilities* to the various diagnostic or treatment options being considered.[9]

The study of how patients view different health outcomes is a fascinating and expanding science which is covered in detail elsewhere.[9,10] Patients are generally stoical about minor side effects of effective interventions but assign greater importance than health professionals to unlikely but potentially serious outcomes. For example, most people with deep venous thrombosis would readily accept a greatly increased risk of a sore leg rather than risk a tiny chance of an intracerebral haemorrhage associated with streptokinase-plus-heparin therapy compared to heparin alone, even though their doctors tend to put the risk–benefit ratio in favour of combination therapy.[11]

Formal decision-analysis, in which the different diagnostic and management options are drawn out like the branches of a probability tree, given numerical values corresponding to their likely benefits and burdens, and multiplied through by personal utilities assigned by the patient,[12] has its advocates and also its opponents. The former argue that medical decision-making based on decision-analysis can unite the potentially conflicting paradigms of evidence-based medicine (the need for clinical interventions to be based on sound research evidence), cost-effective medicine (the need for the choice of intervention to take account of financial cost) and preference-driven medicine (the need for interventions to incorporate the values and preferences of both the individual patient and the wider society).[13] Opponents of the decision-analysis approach, however, argue that the "probability tree" model is unreliable, reductionist, and gives a false objectivity to decisions which are ultimately intuitive and highly context-dependent,[14] and that in any case, such time-consuming calculations rarely influence decision-making in practice.[15]

In the light of these arguments,[16] we describe below four situations, arising in our own work as general practitioners, which may assist in demonstrating the role of a context-sensitive approach to evidence-based practice. Although based on real clinical problems, certain details have been changed to protect the confidentiality of our patients.

Case 1: A 54-year-old woman with atypical chest "pain"

The story of Mrs Ahmed is shown in Figure 5.1. Using Pendleton's task-orientated model[2] as modified by Sullivan and MacNaughton,[4] the role of evidence in the management of this patient is not easy to spot. Mrs Ahmed's likely condition has been well described anecdotally and explored qualitatively.[17] In an ideal world, this qualitative evidence would be supplemented by epidemiological data on the prognostic accuracy of the patient's unusual and apparently classical history, and comparative studies of different management strategies. But, as is often the case with transcultural medical problems, quantitative evidence to guide diagnostic, prognostic and therapeutic decisions is simply not available.

The general practitioner is faced with a distressed patient who has placed a particular interpretation on her symptoms, and a negative physical examination. Clinical judgement says that the pre-test likelihood of organic disease is small, and hence both the diagnostic usefulness and the cost-effectiveness of further investigations will probably be low, although Mrs Ahmed's smoking status, serum cholesterol level and other coronary risk factors should be given consideration.[18,19] Standard prognostic data collected on patients from a different cultural background would suggest that the pre-test probability of organic coronary artery disease is 3.2% in an asymptomatic individual, 8.4% in "non-anginal chest pain" and 32% in "atypical angina".[20] Whilst a normal resting ECG is extremely reassuring when the patient presents with the symptoms suggesting a myocardial infarction in the emergency room,[21] its value in assessing the full range of acute chest pain syndromes is less clear cut.[22] In most cases, a resting ECG would neither rule in nor rule out the diagnosis.[20,23] Standard advice would be "do not test [with an ECG], and do not treat" but, again using clinical judgement rather than objective research evidence, the doctor decides that the utility of a normal ECG result in reassuring this particular patient will be high. Furthermore, an ECG is relatively cheap, non-invasive and unlikely to produce adverse reactions.

If she orders a resting ECG, however, the doctor should do so in the knowledge that its sensitivity for excluding organic pathology is low, and she should recognise the danger of having a falsely negative test for ischaemic heart disease filed in the notes. Another approach, which the purists may prefer, is to present Mrs Ahmed with the truth – that ruling out organic heart disease has been done on the basis of the history and clinical examination, and that, because an ECG is unlikely substantially to alter this decision, the investigation is not indicated. Such an approach may cause the patient short-term distress and produce conflict in the consultation, but may ultimately lead to greater mutual trust and more informed decision-making by this patient in the future.[24]

Case 2: Screening for Down's syndrome using the triple serum test

Shirley Booth is a 34-year-old primary-school teacher who is 14 weeks pregnant. She has a 10-year-old son, Robin, and has been trying for a second child for 8 years; she miscarried 2 years ago at 11 weeks and found it deeply upsetting. The community midwife has booked her for delivery at the local hospital and mentioned "a blood test for Down's syndrome". Mrs Booth asks you "Should I have the test, Doctor?"

The decision to advise a patient whether or not to undergo a particular screening test may, at first sight, seem less dependent on research evidence than advising them to take medication or have an operation. It is true that whereas new drug treatments are closely scrutinised by the Committee for the Safety of Medicines in the UK before being granted a licence, there is no equivalent procedure for diagnostic and screening tests. Yet many such tests have the potential to do harm – either directly, for example internal bleeding caused by liver biopsy, or indirectly, by arousing anxiety, particularly following a false-positive test.[25]

Having a blood test in early pregnancy is a routine experience, and very few women are even told they are being tested for conditions such as syphilis. The blood test for Down's syndrome, however, has far-reaching implications. In order to help Mrs Booth make an informed decision on whether to have the test, you need to consider a number of questions from her perspective:

(1)   *"What is my risk of having a Down's syndrome baby?"*

The risk of a Down's syndrome pregnancy in a woman of 34 is about 1 in 500.[26]

(2)   *"What exactly does the screening test involve?"*

In some districts, the test routinely offered to pregnant women uses the levels of three chemical markers in the blood – α-fetoprotein (AFP), human chorionic gonadotrophin (HCG) and unconjugated oestriol (E3). These are combined with the woman's age and the gestational age of the fetus in a computer program to give an estimate of her personal risk (such as 1 in 100 or 1 in 2000) of having a Down's syndrome baby. The test does *not* tell her that the fetus she is carrying does or does not have Down's syndrome. This is an important point that is not always grasped either by health professionals or by the patients they advise.[27]

(3)   *"What does it mean if the test is positive?"*

The test is usually expressed as "higher than normal risk" (test positive) or "not higher than normal risk" (test negative). The cut-off point for defining "normal risk" varies from laboratory to laboratory but is commonly set at a risk of 1 in 250. Some laboratories will give the actual figure for the patient's individual risk. It is, of course, a somewhat paternalistic decision to define an acceptable or "normal" level of risk for a particular outcome, but similar decisions are routine in clinical practice – for example, when considering whether to treat mild hypertension or hypercholesterolaemia.

(4)   *"So a positive test means that my baby might have Down's syndrome, and a negative test means I'm OK – is that right?"*

The triple test will pick up 50–60% of Down's syndrome fetuses.[28] Conversely, 40–50% of fetuses with Down's syndrome will be missed by serum screening (i.e. the test will be negative despite the condition being present). This kind of statistic is of value to epidemiologists, purchasing authorities and planners, but will be of little use to Mrs Booth, who is likely to want to know with what degree of certainty a positive or negative test result will tell her that *her* baby does or does not have Down's syndrome. In the language of the epidemiologists, these chances are expressed respectively as the *positive predictive value (PPV)* and *negative predictive value (NPV)* of the test.[29]

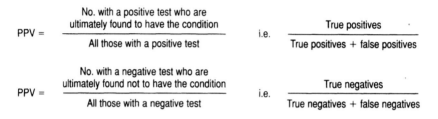

Note that both these values will vary according to the cut-off used to define "normal risk". Using a cut-off of 1 in 250, the PPV of the triple test in women under 35 is 1 in 38 – i.e. once she has tested positive, Mrs Booth has a 1 in 38 chance of having a baby with Down's syndrome.[28] Another value which Mrs Booth will probably want to know is her chance of carrying a Down's syndrome baby even if her test is negative. This is calculated as "1 – NPV" and is approximately 1 in 1900.[29-31]

The different perspectives of patients and health professionals in relation to antenatal screening tests are discussed in detail by Wendy Farrant and Jo Green.[32,33] In general, patients have the test to confirm that they are "OK" (i.e. to demonstrate *absence* of disease), but doctors design the tests to detect the *presence* of disease. Thus, patients are, in general, more interested in the NPV of the test than the PPV. This may seem a subtle distinction but it is critical in the discussion with Mrs Booth.

(5) *"What do I do if my test comes back positive?"*

The screening test results may take 2 weeks to arrive. If her result is positive, she will be offered a more definitive test, amniocentesis, which has an almost 100% PPV and NPV.[34] However, amniocentesis is associated with an increased risk of miscarriage – 1% above the baseline rate of 0.7% after 16 weeks.[34] This means that with a cut-off for "normal risk" placed at 1 in 250, serum screening will lead to the loss of 50% as many chromosomally normal babies as it will detect Down's syndrome babies.

It is at this point in the discussion that Mrs Booth's feelings and preferences (sometimes referred to as her *utilities*) must be considered. She is a teacher and may well have had personal experience of Down's syndrome children. This might lead her to feel that such a child would be much loved and she could cope, or conversely that she and her family could not cope with a child with special needs.

It took her 6 years to get pregnant and that pregnancy 2 years ago ended in miscarriage. She may consider that increasing her chance of miscarriage by 1% is not acceptable. This aspect of the discussion must be tackled sensitively – about 20% of women who test positive on serum screening decline amniocentesis.[35] What if Mrs Booth held strong religious views and would not accept termination, or lived in an area (such as Northern Ireland) where abortion was not an option? She might, nevertheless, wish to know about her baby to prepare herself and her family emotionally and practically. Should she be denied the test because it does not alter *our* management? It alters hers.

Other possible areas for discussion with her are given below.

- What are the advantages and disadvantages of going straight for amniocentesis rather than building in a delay whilst awaiting serum screening results? (25% of women over 35 will be advised to have amniocentesis after serum screening.[36])?
- Is an ultrasound scan necessary to give an accurate estimate of the gestational age of the fetus? (The answer is probably yes.[31])
- Can an antenatal ultrasound scan itself accurately detect Down's syndrome, thus avoiding the increased risk of miscarriage with amniocentesis? (The answer is probably not in the general antenatal population using current standard equipment, although more sensitive scans undertaken in specialised units in the first trimester offer considerable hope for a more accurate and less invasive test in the future.[37,38])

The different options open to Mrs Booth are summarised in decision tree format in Figure 5.2, which has been constructed from a number of sources.[26,28,29] Mrs Booth needs time, to think about the options open to her, discuss them with her husband and maybe return with him to talk to you further. She needs to understand the implications of the result of the test and know how and when she will receive this result. The person passing on the result also needs to know these implications and avoid stating simply that her test is "normal" or "abnormal". Written information about the nature of the screening test and the meaning of the results generally leads to greater satisfaction with the test.[25]

In the end Mrs Booth finds that the prospect of holding herself responsible for a miscarriage is too awful and she declines serum screening. She has a healthy boy 6 months later who is chromosomally normal. Remember that even without screening tests, we knew that the odds of this outcome were 99.8% (see question (1) above).[26] Many other women in comparable circumstances would have decided in favour of the test.

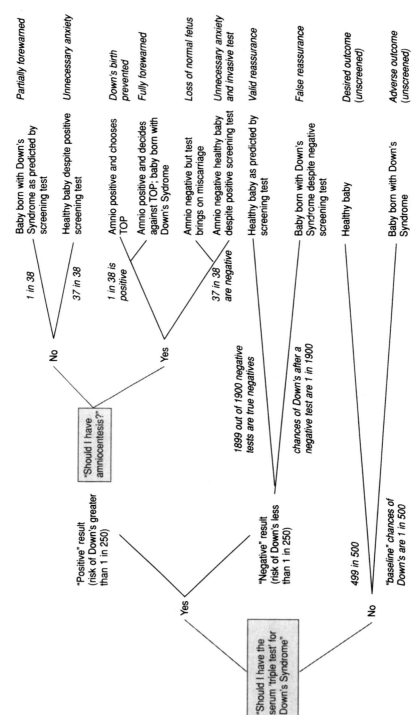

Fig 5.2 Options to be considered by a 34-year-old woman contemplating serum screening for Down's syndrome

Whilst at the time of writing the triple test is still the most widely used screening test for Down's syndrome in the UK, other potentially more accurate tests are being developed and the numerical values in the first decision node in Figure 5.2 may soon improve in the patient's favour.[39] If you are interested in developing a more sophisticated decision tree approach to complex clinical situations such as this one, see an interesting article by van der Meulen and colleagues[40] – screening for Down's syndrome is used to illustrate the possibility of assigning a number to the "disutility" ("bad experience" factor) of different patient outcomes.

Case 3: A 67-year-old man with non-rheumatic atrial fibrillation

Henry Rawlinson is a 67-year-old retired gamekeeper. Six months ago he had a transient ischaemic attack (TIA) which involved his right arm and the right side of his face. He recovered within a few hours. Today he has come to see you because of pain in his chest which you decide is muscular. You examine him and find that he is normotensive, with no signs of valvular heart disease, but is in atrial fibrillation (AF). You could now discuss reducing his risk of future stroke.

If you have access to the Cochrane Library on disk or CD-ROM, and we strongly recommend that you do, you can access the Cochrane Database of Systematic Reviews (CDSR), search for "fibrillation" and find, at the time of writing, 14 systematic reviews, three of which are concerned with secondary stroke prevention in patients with non-rheumatic AF.[41-43] All three reviews are based on the same randomised prospective multicentre study of secondary prevention in non-rheumatic atrial fibrillation after transient ischaemic attack or minor stroke.[44]

As in the previous case (and the one which follows), the first question to ask from the patient's perspective is:

What is my risk of stroke if I have no treatment?

One of the relevant Cochrane reviews shows that the prognosis of patients in AF, with a history of cerebral ischaemia is poor: after an initial stroke or TIA, there is a 2–15% (depending on the study) risk of recurrence in the first year, and a 2–5% annual risk thereafter if no prophylaxis is given.[41]

A number of options are open to Mr Rawlinson:

- He could take an antiplatelet (low) dose of aspirin – i.e. 75–300 mg daily. In a randomised prospective trial against no therapy,[44] 300 mg of aspirin was shown to prevent up to 40 vascular events (mainly strokes) per 1000 users per year, a 16% reduction in risk. In this trial, aspirin was also associated with nine major bleeds per 1000, compared with seven amongst controls – i.e. two extra bleeds per 1000 users per year.

- He could take anticoagulant therapy such as warfarin. Effective anticoagulation approximately halves the risk of recurrence compared to aspirin therapy, and reduces it by two-thirds compared to placebo,[42] preventing up to 90 vascular events per 1000 users per year. However, it increases the risk of major bleeds by 21 per 1000 (none of these bleeds was intracerebral).

Note that although Koudstaal's reviews were recently amended in 1999, the trials included were both secondary care studies co-ordinated from teaching hospitals. You would be wise to check for more recent randomised controlled trials, especially those conducted in primary care. A search of the MEDLINE database at the time of writing revealed no further completed studies, but it did reveal an ongoing large multicentre study of warfarin against aspirin and a dipyridamole/aspirin combination, whose results will be available in a few years' time.[45] In addition, a recent meta-analysis confirms the conclusions of Koudstaal's review,[46] and an accompanying editorial argues persuasively that anticoagulation is particularly beneficial in the elderly and those with a past history of cerebrovascular events – simply because of the higher baseline risk of this group.[47]

With these figures, Mr Rawlinson is in a better position to make a decision about prevention. He lives 10 miles from the surgery and 3 miles up a track on the edge of a forest. Coming for his weekly blood tests will be difficult for him (or for you if he has no transport!) and he would rather not take tablets at all. However, he is extremely keen to prevent a serious stroke. In the end he decides (with your help) that the evidence suggests that *for patients like him*, there is a worthwhile advantage in taking warfarin rather than aspirin with his current clinical risk profile. Both you and he will await the results of ongoing research with interest.

(Incidentally, your review of treatment options for secondary stroke prevention in a patient with non-rheumatic atrial fibrillation would not be complete without consideration of remedies other than the use of anticoagulants and aspirin – see the Cochrane database for further details of management – for example, by means of lipid lowering or antioxidants.)

Case 4: A 58-year-old man with asymptomatic hypertension

Mr Hugh Clayton, a 55-year-old white businessman, had visited the doctor six times in his entire life. On this occasion, he had a twisted ankle. He was seen by the practice nurse, who checked his blood pressure opportunistically and found it to be 214/122 mmHg. Subsequent readings taken under standard recommended conditions[48] were 196/98, 188/102 and 168/96 (average of these three readings 184/98). He was a slim non-smoker who walked 4 miles every day. Routine enquiry revealed no relevant family history (both parents and three siblings were alive and well). Standard investigations, including random plasma glucose level, renal function and a resting ECG, were normal. His fasting plasma cholesterol level was 4.8 mmol/l.

Diagnosing and managing essential hypertension is perceived by many family doctors to be a mundane and uncontroversial task – so much so that the key steps of evidence-based practice (defining the problem, formulating an important and answerable clinical question, searching the literature, interpreting the evidence and applying the intervention) seem to border on overkill. But clinicians who approach the secondary literature (i.e. reviews, meta-analyses, guidelines, etc.) with searching questions on this subject of hypertension will find the current recommendations evidence burdened rather than evidence-based.[49] Guidelines and protocols on the management of hypertension abound,[48,50,51] all based on the same primary research evidence, yet they conflict markedly with one another when applied to real patients in practice.[52] This is largely due to the fact that guideline writers tend to be "experts" in the clinical management of the condition in question rather than in the interpretation of research evidence. In particular, they may fail to undertake a full systematic review of the literature or fail to distinguish absolute from relative risk.[53] With our hypothetical patient in mind, let us explore the evidence ourselves.

Questions about Mr Clayton's prognosis if untreated (what would happen if his blood pressure remained at this level?) or treated (what would happen if it were successfully lowered by around 10 mmHg?) can be answered confidently in terms of "*relative* risk reduction" (Figure 5.3): treatment would be associated with reduction of one-quarter to one-third of the risk of major cardiovascular events.[54] But this begs the question: "what *is* this baseline risk of major cardiovascular events?". After all, a RRR of one-third could be referring to the reduction of a 1 in 700 000 risk to 1 in 1 000 000 at the expense of fatigue, postural dizziness, nocturia, impaired glucose tolerance, gout and impotence, to say nothing of the anxiety generated by offering an asymptomatic individual the mantle of the sick role![55] However, a one-third relative risk reduction could also refer to a 1 in 7 risk being reduced to about 1 in 10. Thus, we see that relative risk reduction following an intervention really needs to be viewed in conjunction with the patient's baseline risk without intervention, in order to determine the significance of any given relative risk reduction. This is expressed as the "*absolute* risk reduction":

Absolute risk reduction (ARR) = CER – EER
Relative risk reduction (RRR) = (CER – EER)/CER
Number needed to treat (NNT) = 1/ARR
CER = control event rate (i.e. rate of major cardiovascular events in the untreated group)
EER = experimental event rate (i.e. rate of major cardiovascular events in the treatment group)

The clinical epidemiologists tell us that the most patient-centred way of interpreting the results of trials on therapy is the number needed to treat (see above), which is the reciprocal of the absolute risk reduction and expresses how many patients would need to receive a particular treatment (such as a drug or operation) to achieve or avoid a particular outcome (cure, death, stroke, etc.).[56] The results of one large study in the UK suggest that around 850 patients with essential hypertension would need to be treated for a year to prevent one stroke.[57] In other words, if around 850 people took no treatment for their high blood pressure, one of them would have a stroke that would otherwise have been avoided.

But as Mr Clayton explained to me, he doesn't care much about that one person in 850 – so long as it isn't him! Glasziou and Irwig have argued that the question of whether to advise a patient to follow a particular treatment is best addressed by assessing the overall potential benefits and risks in that individual patient and not by recourse to the inclusion and exclusion criteria of the trial that demonstrated the treatment's efficacy.[58] Whereas the benefit from a preventive therapy increases with an individual's risk of the condition being prevented, the incidence of adverse reactions is relatively constant across all risk groups. Hence, for all treatments there is a level of risk at which the potential adverse effects outweigh the possible benefits.[59]

To assess Mr Clayton's overall risk of cardiovascular disease events, we need to look at more than just his blood pressure. Epidemiological observations such as the Framingham study have demonstrated that the major risk factors of smoking, left ventricular hypertrophy, hypercholesterolaemia and glucose intolerance all multiply the risk of stroke, such that a 55-year-old man with all these risk factors (the "high risk" patient in Figure 5.3) has 10–15 times the risk of stroke at any given

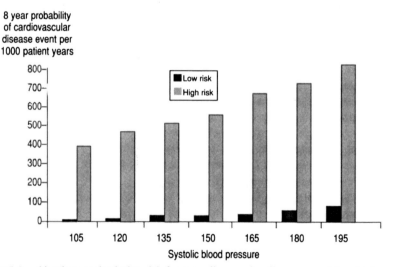

Fig 5.3 Absolute and relative risk for a cardiovascular disease event in a high- and low-risk 55-year-old man by systolic blood pressure.[61]

level of systolic blood pressure compared with a man of the same age with no additional risk factors (the "low risk" individual in Figure 5.3).[60]

As Alderman has shown, the results of intervention trials such as the UK Medical Research Council (MRC) Working Party Trial of Mild Hypertension support the approach of a sliding scale of treatment threshold based on risk stratification.[61] Untreated, a systolic blood pressure above 160 mmHg was associated in this trial with a risk of cardiovascular events of 3.7 to 149 per 1000 over an 8-year period, depending on the presence or absence of other risk factors. In treated patients, antihypertensive medication produced NNTs that varied from 20 to 1000, depending on age and the presence of hypercholesterolaemia, obesity, smoking and ischaemic changes on the ECG.[62] An approach to cardiovascular risk management in which treatment was based on thresholds of absolute risk rather than the level of any single risk factor would save more lives while exposing fewer people to the inconvenience of drug treatment.[63]

Let us return to Mr Clayton, our hypothetical patient with the isolated risk factor of hypertension. He is able and willing to participate in the decision about how to manage his problem. What he needs from his general practitioner, then, is an estimate of his likely risk of avoidable morbidity if he chooses not to take medication. Whilst this risk cannot be quantified exactly, the patient's lack of additional risk factors suggests that it lies closer to the 3.7 per 1000 over 8 years, in the lowest risk subgroup of the MRC trial, than to the 149 per 1000 in the highest risk subgroup. Reference to tables of risk stratification available on the Internet, such as the New Zealand Guidelines for Hypertension Management,[64] suggest that Mr Clayton's absolute risk of developing a cardiovascular disease event over 5 years lies between 5% and 10%, and that 25–50 people like him would need to be treated for this period to prevent one event.

Mr Clayton decided, on balance, that he did not wish to take tablets at this stage, a reflection of his personal utilities for the risks and benefits of drug therapy. Note that a different patient with the same risk profile who is presented with the same outcome odds might choose to start on a tablet immediately. This apparent inconsistency is exactly what patient-centred application of evidence is all about. Note also that balancing the risks and benefits of antihypertensive drug treatment in today's consultation (appraising the evidence) is a small aspect of the general practitioner's overall responsibility towards Mr Clayton, which may include a similar assessment of non-drug treatments (such as taking regular exercise, reducing alcohol intake and following a low-salt diet), pushing home the educational message that dangerously high blood pressure may remain asymptomatic and that (say) 3-monthly review is therefore essential, and, as Figure 5.1 demonstrates, nurturing the therapeutic relationship necessary for productive dialogue and informed consent for future decisions about this patient's health.

Conclusion

In these four examples, we have tried to show you how research-based evidence – from the descriptive sociological study to the systematic review of randomised trials – can aid decision-making in the primary care consultation. In writing this chapter, we found that some relevant evidence (such as a Cochrane review on secondary prevention of stroke) was easy to access and interpret, but we spent many hours searching databases and medical libraries for answers to seemingly straightforward clinical questions (such as the prognosis of untreated mild hypertension or the negative predictive value of the triple test for Down's syndrome). Time is not on the side of the busy GP or nurse practitioner, and we hope that over the next few years, the vital task of tracking down and making readily accessible this type of patient-centred evidence will be addressed by the co-ordinated efforts of academic institutions, health authorities and patient organisations.

As Sackett and colleagues have rightly pointed out, evidence-based medicine is not cook-book medicine with predetermined, inflexible "recipes" for managing patients.[65] Contrary to popular belief, neither does it subjugate the "art" of medicine (sensitivity to the personal circumstances and priorities of the individual patient) to the "science" of large-scale clinical trials and surveys. On the contrary, judicious use of the best available evidence *requires* the primary care practitioner to spend time both listening and explaining to the patient – who is, after all, the real expert on his or her physical, mental and social circumstances.[66] As one of us has argued elsewhere, the "evidence" of evidence-based medicine is necessarily derived from rigorous research on distant populations, but the *application* of this evidence in the clinical context requires detailed attention to the patient's unique personal story – hence, "evidence-based" and "narrative-based" medicine (the "science" and the "art" of clinical practice) are not mutually exclusive approaches but two sides of the same coin.[67] Given that the values and preferences of the individual patient can preclude certain management options, our time will often be better spent establishing this perspective than combing the libraries in search of evidence that will ultimately prove irrelevant.

Acknowledgement

We would like to thank Professor Howard Cuckle for his help with part of this chapter.

References

1 Slawson DC, Shaughnessy AF, Bennett JH. Becoming a medical information master: feeling good about not knowing everything. *J Fam Pract* 1994;5:505–13.

2 Pendleton D, Schofield T, Take P, Havelock P. *The consultation: an approach to learning and teaching*. Oxford: Oxford University Press, 1987.

3 Byrne PS, Long BFL. *Doctors talking to patients*. London: HMSO, 1976.

4 Sullivan FM, MacNaughton RJ. Evidence in consultations: interpreted and individualised. *Lancet* 1996;348:941–3.

5 Sackett DL, Haynes RB, Guyatt GH, Tugwell P. *Clinical epidemiology – a basic science for clinical medicine*. London: Little, Brown & Co., 1991, pp 305–33.

6 Hope T. *Evidence-based patient choice. Report to the Anglia and Oxford Regional Health Authority into the use of evidence-based information for enhancing patient choice*. Oxford: University of Oxford, October 1995.

7 Naylor CD. Grey zones of clinical practice: some limits to evidence-based medicine. *Lancet* 1995;345:840–2.

8 Haynes RB, Hayward RSA, Lomas J. Bridges between health care evidence and clinical practice. *J Am Informatics Assoc* 1995;2:342–50.

9 Mehrez A, Gafni A. Quality-adjusted life-years, utility theory and healthy years equivalents. *Med Decision Making* 1989;9:142–9.

10 Kassirer JK. Incorporating patients' preferences into medical decisions. *New Engl J Med* 1994;330:1895–6.

11 O'Meara JJ III, McNutt RA, Evans AT, Moore SW, Downs SM. A decision analysis of streptokinase plus heparin as compared with heparin alone for deep-vein thrombosis. *New Engl J Med* 1994;330:1864–9.

12 Thornton JG, Lilford RJ, Johnson N. Decision analysis in medicine. *BMJ* 1992;302:1099–103.

13 Dowie J. "Evidence-based", "cost-effective", and "preference-driven" medicine. *J Health Serv Res Policy* 1996;1:104–13.

14 Asch DA, Herschey JC. Why some health policies don't make sense at the bedside. *Ann Intern Med* 1995;122:846–50.

15 Poses RM, Cebul RD, Wigton RS. You can lead a horse to water – improving physicians' knowledge of probabilities may not affect their decisions. *Med Decision Making* 1995;15:65–75.

16 Greenhalgh T. Is my practice evidence-based? *BMJ* 1996;313:957–8.

17 Krause I-B. Sinking heart – a Punjabi communication of distress. *Soc Sci Med* 1989;29:563–75.

18 Sackett DL, Haynes RB, Guyatt GH, Tugwell P. *Clinical epidemiology – a basic science for clinical medicine*. London: Little, Brown & Co., 1991, pp 69–152.

19 Bennett NM, Greenland P. Coronary Artery Disease. In: Panzer PJ, Black ER, Griner PF, eds. *Diagnostic strategies for common medical problems*. Philadelphia: American College of Physicians, 1991.

20 Bennett NM, Greenland P. Coronary Artery Disease. In: Panzer PJ, Black ER, Griner PF, eds. *Diagnostic strategies for common medical problems*. Philadelphia: American College of Physicians, 1991, p. 46.

21 Savonitto S, Ardissino D, Granger CB, *et al*. Prognostic value of the admission electrocardiogram in acute coronary syndromes [see comments]. *JAMA* 1999;281:707–13.

22 Zalenski RJ, McCarren M, Roberts R, *et al*. An evaluation of a chest pain diagnostic protocol to exclude acute cardiac ischemia in the emergency department. *Arch Intern Med* 1997;157:1085–91.

23 Pozen MW, D'Agostino RB, Selker HP, *et al*. A predictive instrument to improve coronary care unit admission practices in acute ischaemic heart disease. *N Engl J Med* 1984;310:1273–82.

24 Coulter A. Partnerships with patients: the pros and cons of shared clinical decision-making. *J Health Serv Res Policy* 1997;2:112–21.

25 Marteau TM, Kidd J, Michie S, *et al.* Anxiety, knowledge and satisfaction in women receiving false positive results on routine prenatal screening: a randomised controlled trial. *J Psychosom Obstet Gynaecol* 1993;14:185–96.

26 Cuckle HS, Wald NJ, Thompson SG. Estimating a woman's risk of having a pregnancy associated with Down's syndrome using her age and alpha-fetoprotein level. *Br J Obstet Gynaecol* 1987;94:387–402.

27 Sadler M. Serum screening for Down's syndrome: how much do health professionals know? *Br J Obstet Gynaecol* 1997;104:176–9.

28 Cuckle H. Established markers in second trimester maternal serum. *Early Human Dev* 1996;47:Suppl S27–S29.

29 Cuckle H, Sehmi I, Holding S. Nomograms to help inform women considering Down's syndrome screening. *Eur J Obstet Gynaecol Reprod Biol* 1996;69:69–72.

30 Wald NJ, Cuckle HS, Densem JW, Kennard A, Smith D. Maternal serum screening for Down's Syndrome: the effect of routine ultrasound scan determination of gestational age and adjustment for maternal weight. *Br J Obstet Gynaecol* 1992;99:144–9.

31 Wald NJ, Kennard A, Densem JW, *et al.* Antenatal maternal serum screening for Down's syndrome: results of a demonstration project. *BMJ* 1992;305:391–4.

32 Green JM, Snowdon C, Statham H. Pregnant women's attitudes to abortion and prenatal screening. *J Reprod Infant Psychol* 11:31–9.

33 Farrant W. "Who's for amniocentesis?" The politics of prenatal screening. In: Homans H, ed. *The sexual politics of reproduction.* London: Gower, 1985.

34 Tabor A, Philip J, Madsen M, *et al.* Randomised controlled trial of genetic amniocentesis in 4606 low-risk women. *Lancet* 1986;1:1287–92.

35 Dick PT. Periodic health examination, 1996 update. 1. Prenatal screening for, and diagnosis of Down Syndrome. *Can Med Assoc J* 1996;154:465–79.

36 Haddow JE, Palomaki GE, Knight GJ, *et al.* Reducing the need for amniocentesis in women 35 years of age or older with serum markers for screening. *N Engl J Med* 1994;330:1114–18.

37 Adekunle O, Gopee A, el-Sayed M, Thilaganathan B. Increased first trimester nuchal translucency: pregnancy and infant outcomes after routine screening for Down's syndrome in an unselected antenatal population. *Br J Radiol* 1999;72:457–60.

38 Thilaganathan B, Sairam S, Michailidis G, Wathen NC. First trimester nuchal translucency: effective routine screening for Down's syndrome. *Br J Radiol* 1999;72:946–8.

39 Haddow JE, Palomaki GE, Knight GJ, Williams J, Miller WA, Johnson A. Screening of maternal serum for fetal Down's syndrome in the first trimester. *New Engl J Med* 1998;338:955–61.

40 van der Meulen JH, Mol BW, Pajkrt E, van Lith JM, Voorn W. Use of the disutility ratio in prenatal screening for Down's syndrome. *Br J Obstet Gynaecol* 1999;106:108–15.

41 Koudstaal PJ. Anticoagulants for preventing stroke in patients with nonrheumatic atrial fibrillation and a history of stroke or transient ischaemic attack (Cochrane Review). In: *Cochrane Collaboration. Cochrane Library,* Issue 3. Oxford: Update Software, 2000.

42 Koudstaal PJ. Anticoagulants versus antiplatelet therapy for preventing stroke in patients with nonrheumatic atrial fibrillation and a history of stroke or transient ischaemic attacks (Cochrane Review). In: *Cochrane Collaboration. Cochrane Library,* Issue 4. Oxford: Update Software, 2000.

43 Koudstaal PJ. Antiplatelet therapy for preventing stroke in patients with

nonrheumatic atrial fibrillation and a history of stroke or transient ischaemic attacks (Cochrane Review). In: *Cochrane Collaboration. Cochrane Library*, Issue 4. Oxford. Update Software, 2000.

44 Secondary prevention in non-rheumatic atrial fibrillation after transient ischaemic attack or minor stroke. EAFT (European Atrial Fibrillation Trial) Study Group. *Lancet* 1993;**342**:1255-62.

45 De Schryver EL. Design of ESPRIT: an international randomized trial for secondary prevention after non-disabling cerebral ischaemia of arterial origin. European/Australian Stroke Prevention in Reversible Ischaemia Trial (ESPRIT) group. *Cerebrovasc Dis* 2000;**10**:147-50.

46 Hart RG, Benavente O, McBride R, Pearce LA. Antithrombotic therapy to prevent stroke in patients with atrial fibrillation: a meta-analysis. *Ann Intern Med* 1999;**131**:492-501.

47 Hart RG, Halperin JL. Atrial fibrillation and thromboembolism: a decade of progress in stroke prevention. *Ann Intern Med* 1999;**131**:688-95.

48 Ramsay LE, Williams B, Johnston GD, *et al.* British Hypertension Society guidelines for hypertension management, 1999: summary. *BMJ* 1999;**319**:630-5.

49 Jackson RT, Sackett DL. Guidelines for managing raised blood pressure. *BMJ* 1996;**313**:64-5.

50 Jackson R, Barham P, Bills J, *et al.* Management of raised blood pressure in New Zealand: a discussion document. *BMJ* 1993;**307**:107-10.

51 Feldman RD, Campbell N, Larochelle P, *et al.* 1999 Canadian recommendations for the management of hypertension. Task Force for the Development of the 1999 Canadian Recommendations for the Management of Hypertension. *Can Med Assoc J* 1999;**161**:Suppl 12: S1-17.

52 Fahey TP, Peters TJ. What constitutes controlled hypertension? Patient based comparison of hypertension guidelines. *BMJ* 1996;**313**:93-6.

53 Jackson R. Guidelines on preventing cardiovascular disease in clinical practice. *BMJ* 2000;**320**:659-61.

54 Gueyffier F, Boutitie F, Boisel J-P, *et al.* Effect of antihypertensive drug treatment on cardiovascular outcomes in women and men: a meta-analysis of individual patient data from randomised controlled trials. *Ann Intern Med* 1997;**126**:761.

55 Haynes RB, Sackett DL, Tayler DW, Gibson ES, Johnson AL. Increased absenteeism from work after detection and labelling of hypertensive patients. *New Engl J Med* 1978;**229**:741-4.

56 Cook RJ, Sackett DL. The number needed to treat: a clinically useful measure of treatment effect. *BMJ* 1995;**310**:452-4.

57 Medical Research Council Working Party. MRC trial of mild hypertension: principal results. *BMJ* 1985;**291**:97-104.

58 Glasziou P, Irwig LM. An evidence-based approach to individualising treatment. *BMJ* 1995;**311**:1356-9.

59 Davey Smith G, Egger M. Who benefits from medical interventions? *BMJ* 1994;**308**:72-4.

60 Kannel WB, Sorlie P. Hypertension in Framingham. In: Paul O, ed. *Epidemiology and control of hypertension*. New York: Stratton, 1975, pp 553-92.

61 Alderman MH. Blood pressure management: individualised treatment based on absolute risk and potential for benefit. *Ann Intern Med* 1993;**119**:329-35.

62 Medical Research Council Working Party. Stroke and coronary heart disease in mild hypertension: risk factors and the value of treatment. *BMJ* 1988;**296**:1565-70.

63 Baker S, Priest P, Jackson R. Using thresholds based on risk of cardiovascular disease to target treatment for hypertension: modelling events averted and number treated. *BMJ* 2000;**320**:680–5.

64 www.cebm.jr2.ox.ac.uk/docs/prognosis/htm

65 Sackett DL, Rosenberg WMC, Gray JAM, Haynes RB, Richardson WS. Evidence-based medicine: what it is and what it isn't. *BMJ* 1996;**312**:71–2.

66 Tuckett D, Boulton M, Olson C, *et al. Meetings between experts: an approach to sharing ideas in medical consultations.* London: Tavistock Publications, 1985.

67 Greenhalgh T. Narrative based medicine: narrative based medicine in an evidence-based world. *BMJ* 1999;**318**:323–5.

6: Screening and diagnostic tests

J ANDRÉ KNOTTNERUS AND RON AG WINKENS

Introduction

Adequate diagnostic decision-making is the key to effective health care. Most health problems presented to the general practitioner (GP) are self-limiting or can be treated fully in the primary care setting. The general practitioner (GP), who is confronted with an unlimited and undifferentiated range of problems, requires properly collected and correctly interpreted diagnostic information in order to select the best and most efficient management pathway, including possible referral to outpatient or hospital care.

In this chapter, first the primary care context of diagnostic decision-making is described, thereby illustrating the need for a specific evidence-based approach in general practice. After a brief review of some basics of diagnostic testing, examples are given of what evidence-based medicine can mean for history taking, physical examination and additional diagnostic testing in general practice. Finally, the gatekeeping GP is analysed in diagnostic terms.

The spectrum of presented health problems

As a consequence of the GP's gatekeeping function, characteristic differences exist between the spectrum of health problems presented to the GP and the medical specialist. Regarding diagnostic decision-making the most relevant differences can be summarised as follows:

- Most problems presented to a GP have not yet been reduced to a specific category. The "problem space" is large, especially in cases of so-called "vague complaints" such as headache, fatigue or low back pain. The specialist sees patients who have usually been preselected by the GP with respect to specialty and diagnostic category.
- Given particular complaints, severe diseases are much less frequent among patients visiting their GP than among those referred to a specialist.[1-3]

- Disorders are usually seen by the GP at an earlier, less developed stage, which makes their recognition more difficult.[1-4]
- A diagnosis is a starting point for prognostic assessment. In general practice, a particular disease will, by and large, have a more favourable prognosis and be more amenable to treatment than in specialist practice, since the more difficult cases are more frequently referred.[5]
- The GP has more prior knowledge of the patients, their social situation and their care-seeking behaviour, and thus has extra points of reference as regards the probability and prognosis of particular disorders, the risks and the patient's preferences.

The described spectrum of presented health problems has important implications for the GP's diagnostic management.

Hypothesis development and "diagnostic breadth"

Confronted with a large problem space, GPs often have to draw up rather general diagnostic hypotheses: inflammation, malignancy, stress, or even as aspecific as organic/non-organic or pathology/no pathology. This assessment is related to probability, severity and expected consequences. Specialists can formulate more specific hypotheses, because of the GP's preparatory work and the formulated reason for referral.

In this context, the GP needs diagnostic approaches with a large diagnostic breadth to be applied before specific hypotheses can be formulated. Thus, a broad spectrum of diagnostic possibilities can be scanned. Questions about general well-being, weight changes and the development of symptoms over time, and tests such as the erythrocyte sedimentation rate often yield essential, though non-specific, information. Time may also be used as a diagnostic tool in cases where non-specific complaints might hide severe disorders but also an innocent, temporary indisposition.

Reducing the problem space using relatively simple, broadly screening methods is also essential for selecting more specific tests that might be indicated. This is especially important since more advanced methods such as cytologic puncturing and gastrointestinal endoscopy are increasingly available as open access tests.

Diagnostic testing

Discrimination

Diagnostic hypotheses can be tested by diagnostic examinations. These include history taking, physical examination and laboratory and other diagnostics, collectively designated as "tests". By application of tests and the interpretation of the results the (estimated) pre-test probability of a certain disease is transformed to the (estimated) post-test probability of that disease, also called the predictive value of the test result.

The test should add clinically relevant information to the pre-test probability. Hence, it is important to use tests with a good "discriminatory power", i.e. yielding clearly different results for people with and without the disease under consideration, or for people with different diseases. Since 100% certainty can rarely be achieved, the aim is to obtain a relevant degree of certainty: a test should achieve a sufficient predictive value to allow the physician to decide whether additional diagnostic and/or therapeutic steps ought to be taken.

The discriminatory power of a diagnostic test is usually characterised by (a) *sensitivity*: the probability of finding an abnormal result in diseased subjects; and (b) *specificity*: the probability of finding a normal result in non-diseased subjects (see also p. 43). Obviously, the discrimination of a test is better if both sensitivity and specificity are closer to 100%. The lower these parameters, the more false-negative and false-positive results can be expected.

Many clinical tests have two outcome levels: someone either has colic or chest pain, or not. In case of a continuous scale (such as diastolic blood pressure) one may choose a cut-off point when the test result is to be used in deciding for or against certain actions such as prescribing a drug or referring to a specialist. Focusing on test results with two outcome levels (positive or negative), the discriminative power of a test can be summarised in the "likelihood ratio". For a positive result LR is defined as:

$$\frac{\text{probability of a positive result in diseased subjects}}{\text{probability of a positive result in healthy subjects}}$$

$$= \frac{\text{sensitivity}}{100\% - \text{specificity}} \; (= \text{LR}+)$$

The negative result also has its likelihood ratio LR−: (100% sensitivity)/specificity, representing, in words, the ratio of the probability of a negative result in diseased subjects and the probability of a negative result in healthy subjects.

Clearly, the discrimination is zero if LR = 1: diseased and healthy subjects will have the same distribution of positive and negative results, and instead of doing the test one might as well toss a coin. This situation, or one approaching it, might occur more often than is commonly thought, for example in frequently used diagnostic tests such as estimated prostate size on rectal examination and some liver function tests.[6,7] As LR+ exceeds 1, the discriminative power increases. This allows various tests to be compared. For example, a history of typical angina pectoris is highly informative (with an LR+ of 115–120), far more so than atypical complaints (LR+ = 14–15).[8]

More sophisticated and invasive tests such as exercise ECG and thallium scintigraphy have LR+ values rarely exceeding 10 and, for making the diagnosis, often add little independent information to the clinical history. Indeed, specific, sophisticated tests need not always provide a higher discrimination than simple symptoms or tests. In the case of thoracic pain its localisation and character, and the question whether it occurs during exertion, are so essential that further tests can be omitted if history taking shows no suspicious results on these points. Pryor et al. found that history taking is more accurate in discriminating patients with or without cardiovascular disease than exercise electrocardiography.[9] This means that GPs should rely more on a thorough history taking and physical examination rather than on diagnostic tests.

The selection of adequate diagnostic tests for common medical problems can be supported by using compiled information on the discriminative power of a large number of tests, such as those published by Panzer et al.[10] and Sox.[11]

Predictive value

The ultimate goal of diagnostic testing is to go from a pre-test probability, via the application of diagnostic tests, to a clearly higher or lower post-test probability, also called the predictive value of a test result. We can distinguish:

- Positive predictive value = the probability of a disease being present if the test result is positive.
- Negative predictive value = the probability of no disease being present if the result is negative (see also Chapters 4 and 5).

This is illustrated in Table 6.1a,[12] showing the possible results of physical examination for ankle fracture in case of ankle trauma. The starting point is a sensitivity for physical examination of 95% and a specificity of 90%.[12] Furthermore, a pre-test probability of 4% of finding a fracture in a case of sprain-like symptomatology in general practice is assumed.[13] To make things easy, the calculations start from a cohort of 1000 subjects examined because of this symptomatology. The table shows that the predictive value of the conclusion "fracture" (i.e. the positive result) after physical examination alone is 28%, while the conclusion "no fracture" (the negative result) has a predictive value of almost 100%. Apparently, a negative result offers sufficient certainty to reassure the patient and to apply conservative treatment, while a positive result necessitates further investigation, for instance an x ray.

The predictive value of a diagnostic test depends on the pre-test probability. Table 6.1b assumes that the pre-test probability of a fracture in a patient with symptoms of a sprained ankle is considerably higher after preselection through referral by the GP, viz. 20%. Assuming that sensitivity and specificity of the physical examination are the same when performed by a specialist, the predictive value of the positive result will be much higher: 70%. The predictive value of the negative result is somewhat lower now, but still very high: 99%. Hence, the mere difference in pre-test probability in favour of the specialist implies that the latter does produce a much higher predictive value for the abnormal result. This might erroneously suggest that the specialist is a better examiner, although the discriminative power of the test is the same for both: $LR+ = 95\%/(100\% - 90\%) = 9.5$.

Table 6.1 Discrimination and predictive values of physical examination for detecting fractures in ankle trauma, using x ray results as a gold standard[12]

a. **Situation** in general practice where the pre-test probability of fracture is low

Conclusion on basis of physical examination	Results of x ray		
	Fracture	No fracture	Total
Fracture	38	96	134
No fracture	2	864	866
Total	40	960	1000

Sensitivity = 38/40 = 95%.
Specificity = 864/960 = 90%.
Predictive value of conclusion "fracture" = 38/134 = 28%.
Predictive value of conclusion "no fracture" = 864/866 = (almost) 100%.
Pre-test probability of fracture = 40/1000 = 4%.

b. **Situation** in specialist practice where the pre-test probability of fracture is higher

Conclusion on basis of physical examination	Results of x ray		
	Fracture	No fracture	Total
Fracture	190	80	270
No fracture	10	720	730
Total	200	800	1000

Sensitivity and specificity as in (a).
Predictive value of conclusion "fracture" = 190/270 = 70%.
Predictive value of conclusion "no fracture" = 720/730 = 99%.
Pre-test probability of fracture = 200/1000 = 20%.

The calculation can be repeated for other pre-test probabilities. If the pre-test probability in the population examined by the specialist is assumed to be 50%, the predictive value of the positive result would be even higher, viz. 90%. However, the predictive value of the negative result has now fallen to 95%. This may be regarded as an unacceptable risk of false-negative conclusions, suggesting that physical diagnostics should in this situation not determine the subsequent actions and might just as well be omitted.

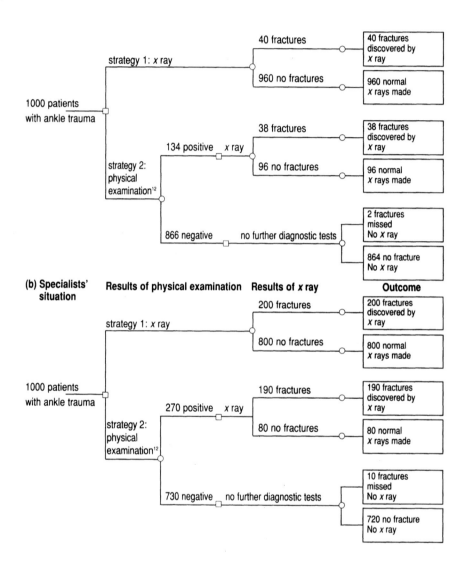

(a) GPs' situation **Results of physical examination** **Results of *x* ray** **Outcome**

(b) Specialists' situation **Results of physical examination** **Results of *x* ray** **Outcome**

Fig 6.1 Decision tree for choosing between strategy 1 (*x* ray for every patient) and strategy 2 (*x* ray only if physical examination yields suspicion of fracture). (Data from Table 6.1)

Evidence based diagnostic decision making

The pre-test probability of diseases is of great importance not only in the interpretation of test results but also in choosing diagnostic strategies. For the example of ankle sprain, Figure 6.1 shows decision trees for choosing between the following strategies:

(I)   The physician orders an x ray for every patient presenting with an ankle trauma.

(II) The physician performs a physical examination in every patient presenting with ankle trauma. x rays are only ordered if the physical examination leads the doctor to suspect a fracture (according to the Ottawa Ankle Rules for example[14]).

The figure is based on cohorts of 1000 subjects with ankle trauma, assuming that the x ray reveals the real situation. The data of Table 6.1 have been inserted into the decision tree: if a GP were to choose strategy I (i.e. complete certainty), this would require 866 extra x rays compared to strategy II in order to detect two extra fractures at first consultation. For the specialist the balance is more favourable: strategy I requires 730 extra x rays to discover 10 extra fractures. The results of each strategy are summarised in Table 6.2.

Table 6.2 Two diagnostic strategies in 1000 patients with ankle trauma

	General practice: pre-test probability of fracture: 4%		Surgeon: pre-test probability of fracture: 20%	
	I	II	I	II
X ray studies	1000	134	1000	270
Fractures detected	40	38	200	190
Fractures missed	0	2	0	10

Strategy I: x ray examination in every case of ankle trauma.
Strategy II: Do a physical examination and x ray only if physical examination yields suspicion of fracture.

Clearly, weighing these strategies requires consideration of the cost-effectiveness in terms of numbers of x rays performed and numbers of extra fractures discovered. Value judgements ("utilities") play a role. One might think of the strain put on the patient (going to the x ray department, radiation load, feeling insecure if no x rays are made, prognosis of a fracture which is not immediately detected); the costs of an x ray; the strain put on the physician (how much blame would attach to him or her if the occasional fracture is missed), etc. In a study by Stiell et al.,[15] the

73

aforementioned Ottawa Ankle Rules resulted in a significant reduction of x rays with no differences in the rate of fractures found.

Applying the concept of "time as a diagnostic tool", the GP can postpone the decision about x rays in doubtful cases. Patients with fractures will still show suspicious symptoms after 5 days, while those without fractures will far less often have symptoms by then. In other words: the sensitivity of physical diagnostics will remain the same while the specificity will increase, implying an increased discrimination. In addition, since a number of patients without fractures will now be free of complaints, the pre-test probability of the remaining symptomatic group has increased. Both strategies will now require fewer x ray studies.

The decision to request tests

In general, tests should only be requested when their results contribute in some way to the diagnostic and/or therapeutic work-up for the individual patient. During a consultation the GP may have come to a certain hypothesis with a greater or lesser degree of certainty. The main reason for diagnostic testing would be to obtain more certainty about the presence or absence of a disease. Additional diagnostic testing is useful when a specific disorder cannot be excluded nor confirmed to a satisfactory level by history and examination. From the doctor's perspective, diagnostic testing is useless when the test results will not change the probability of disease significantly or when they will not influence the work-up for the individual patient. Disease probability cannot be changed dramatically when it is already very high or very low. When, on the basis of complaints, signs and symptoms, the pre-test probability of a particular disease is very low, the GP can be virtually certain that the patient is not ill. Further testing will not change this. A negative test result (which is very likely) can only confirm what is already known, while a positive test result would be very likely to be false-positive. This illustrates the concept of "diagnostic threshold". Below this threshold diagnostic testing is useless. Would it be useful to search for a possible Epstein–Barr viral infection when a patient aged 40 years suffers from fever and sore throat? There is little chance that the patient has mononucleosis. However, would you rely on the normal findings at physical examination when a 60-year-old woman consulted you because she had felt a small lump in her breast? Would you be satisfied with a negative cervical smear in a 41-year-old woman with five children, contact and intermenstrual bleeding and an eroded cervix?

In these latter examples there is, also on the basis of complaints, signs and symptoms, a high probability that the patient is ill. Further testing will not change this. An abnormal test result (which is very likely) can only confirm what is already known and the patient will be treated (if possible) for this disorder. This decision will not be influenced by additional testing

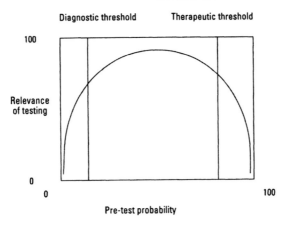

Fig 6.2 The influence of pre-test probability on the relevance of diagnostic testing.

since a negative test result would probably be false-negative. Here, the concept "therapeutic threshold" comes in: beyond this threshold GPs often refer a patient immediately without the risk of any delay eventually emanating from requesting tests first. Think, for example of the middle-aged woman who you strongly suspect to have cervical cancer. One should probably refer immediately without awaiting or even taking a cervical smear. Would you act differently when the test result would be normal?

When the pre-test probability is between the diagnostic and the therapeutic threshold, it is often relevant to perform or request additional diagnostic tests. Figure 6.2 shows these thresholds and their relation to the relevance of testing is visualised.

Consequences of incorrect test use

In an ideal world, GPs should request tests only when this leads to less uncertainty about the expected disorder, they should choose tests with the highest validity and omit other tests that have a higher risk of false-negative or false-positive results.

The inappropriate and excessive use of diagnostic tests can have a number of effects on different levels. On doctor level, as a paradox, it may cause a false certainty. A negative effect on quality of care can not be ruled out. The GP may draw a false conclusion not justified by test characteristics. Simply by using "normal" values as cut-off levels, the risk of a false-positive test result is generally 5% (5% is chosen according to the common assumption that among healthy people 95% will have a normal (laboratory) test result, implying that the probability of a (false) abnormal result is 5%; that is, a specificity of 95%). In case 10 tests are ordered, the risk of at least one false-positive test result has increased to 40%! The probability of at least one false-positive result = 1 − the probability that all test results are normal. For x tests with a specificity of 0.95, this is: $1 - 0.95^x$. For $x = 1$ this is: $1 - 0.95^1 = 0.05$. For $x = 10$ this is: $1 - 0.95^{10} = 0.401$.

Several blood tests are known to have a low validity. If every patient with, for example, a positive Rose–Waaler test was treated as having rheumatoid arthritis, not considering the possibility of a false-positive test result, this would lead to inappropriate referrals and overtreatment. This may lead to somatisation, additional (and afterwards unnecessary) diagnostic testing and adverse effects on patient outcome. Overall, on health care level the sum of all these side-effects is a waste of health care resources leading to unnecessarily high health care expenses.

Therefore, the benefits of evidence-based diagnostic testing in daily practice are clear. Often there is fear of an underutilisation of tests resulting in doctors' delay in diagnosis. However, in research no such effect was found.[16,17] For example, lowered use of diagnostic tests by GPs did not result in increased referrals at a later stage.[17] While each GP is confronted regularly with patients insisting on diagnostic testing, the poor validity of many tests can be used in negotiating with patients about their request. For patients, this can be an eye-opener.

How strong is the evidence base for choosing tests?

If, based on the aforementioned considerations, one decides to request diagnostic tests, the next step would be to select the most appropriate (combination of) test(s). The principles of medical decision-making can help once again. The GP should ask him/herself why diagnostic tests are needed. Are they needed to exclude or to confirm the presence of a disorder? The exclusion or confirmation of a disorder calls for specific test characteristics. For excluding a disorder the GP must rely on a negative test result. False-negative test results should not occur. In other words, the test should be highly sensitive. This means a high sensitivity of the test. The confirmation of a disorder requires a test with a minimal risk of false-positive results and therefore a high specificity.

Unfortunately, for many tests those characteristics are unknown. Moreover, data on test characteristics depend on the situation in which they are assessed.[4] Over the last decades, research on test characteristics has increasingly been attracting attention. However, the inclusion of patients in such studies is quite time consuming in primary care compared to similar studies in specialist care. In hospital care, patients who meet inclusion criteria are much more easy to identify and to monitor, due to the preselection by GPs. Only those patients with a higher pre-test probability are referred to a hospital. As a consequence, most studies on test characteristics are performed in the hospital setting, using a preselected group of patients as study participants. It is because of this same preselection by GPs that the data stemming from such studies cannot be extrapolated to primary care.[18] How sensitive is a test in primary care for patients seeking help in an early phase of a disorder when sensitivity of this test is determined in a hospital setting on patients included in the study in a later, and possibly more pronounced phase of their disorder? How reliable are such tests if they are performed in a primary care setting, or used as near patient tests? Do quality control data from hospital laboratories represent the situation in primary care? The awareness that data on test characteristics from studies in specialist care need not be valid for primary care has led to a growing number of studies assessing test characteristics in primary care. A few examples of such studies follow.

One of the complaints for which patients do consult their GP most frequently is fatigue. In most cases this complaint has no somatic origin. Nevertheless, fatigue has for years been one of the major reasons to search for the presence of anaemia. The test directly related to anaemia, haemoglobin, is one of the most frequently requested tests in primary care. However, in one study no correlation between fatigue and the haemoglobin concentration in a primary care setting was found.[19]

Another test frequently used in primary care is the erythrocyte sedimentation rate (ESR). It has been shown that for patients presenting with a new problem in primary care, ESR is a good test to rule out disorders such as inflammatory diseases relatively confidently.[20] The negative predictive value was 91%, taking 12 mm/hr for men and 28 mm/hr for women as upper limits. This means that pathology can be ruled out for 91% of such patients when the ESR is within normal range. One might, however, question whether this is enough to rely on when it concerns a potentially life-threatening but curable disorder. However, a raised ESR does not necessarily mean that the patient is ill. Overall, 52% of such patients are healthy. This may lead to the conclusion that ESR is a useful test for excluding illness in general in patients with common complaints of short duration; for diagnosing any severe illness ESR is not appropriate.[20]

Another study evaluated the characteristics of several tests involved in the diagnosis of urinary tract infections (UTI). Painful and/or frequent micturition in women 12–65 years of age represents a classical situation in which diagnostic testing should be performed on the basis of the level of pre-test probability. Here, the probability for UTI is 60–65%. Hence, a UTI cannot be confirmed nor excluded solely on the basis of complaints by the patients. Examination of a urine sample is necessary. In earlier studies it was found that urine tests, nitrite testing and the sediment in particular, were reliable tests for confirming/excluding a UTI, with specificity and positive predictive value at times higher than 95%.[21] These were data from studies in laboratory situations. Under practice conditions, however, the same test characteristics were lower and they concluded that urine tests performed under such conditions do not substantially increase the level of certainty on the presence/absence of UTI. GPs should not rely on urine test results, unless urine testing is performed strictly according to optimal standard procedures.[22]

Disseminating knowledge on evidence-based diagnostic management

Simply publishing the results of research on test characteristics in a journal is usually not sufficient to have them applied in daily care. In literature, a variety of methods to disseminate knowledge on test characteristics and a proper use of diagnostic tests have been described. They vary from voluntary methods such as books, literature or postgraduate education to methods confronting doctors with their performance through peer review, feedback and computer reminders or even obligatory methods such as recertification. Studies on such intervention methods have shown that they offer possibilities to disseminate knowledge on test characteristics and the value of principles of evidence-based medicine. Audit and feedback have proven effective means to implement previously set guidelines (for further discussion see Chapter 9). Repeated individual feedback on the appropriateness of test requests of GPs, for example, leads to a substantial and long lasting reduction of inappropriate test requests.[23] The comments to individual GPs can be based on principles of evidence-based medicine, such as "For estimating renal function it is sufficient to have a determination of serum creatinine; adding serum urea testing is not necessary since the sensitivity and specificity of serum urea for renal failure is much lower than that of serum creatinine".

There is growing evidence from literature that computer reminder systems are also an effective way to implement the principles of evidence-based diagnostic testing and to change test ordering behaviour accordingly[24,25] (see also Chapter 8).

Guidelines on diagnostic testing should not only discuss the value of (a variety of) individual tests, but they should also in general focus on the basic principles of evidence-based medicine and medical decision-making. Self-directed learners can learn from distributed guidelines. It is experienced, however, that simply introducing guidelines usually is not enough. The saying of Samuel Johnson remains true: "men more frequently need to be reminded than informed".

The gatekeeping function, the GP as equilibrist

The principle of evidence-based diagnostic testing can also be applied to "the gatekeeping GP" as an overall diagnostic test . One of the most important skills for the GP is differentiating between patients who need further examination, treatment or referral and those who do not. At present, the GP deals with 85–90% of the presented episodes of illness without referral. It is of vital importance that the GP's gatekeeping function is not unjustly discredited. Let us elaborate a hypothetical example. In Table 6.3a it can be seen that of the patients with a particular complaint X who were in need of specialised treatment, the GPs did refer 90% without undue delay: the sensitivity of their referral behaviour is 90%. Ten per cent of the patients with complaint X who did not need specialised treatment were nevertheless referred: the specificity of the referral behaviour is 100% – 10% = 90%. This results in a likelihood ratio of 90%/(100% – 90%) = 9. The GP does achieve a fairly high discrimination, if these figures are compared to those of many individual diagnostic tests.

Table 6.3 The general practitioner's gatekeeping function: referral behaviour of GPs in relation to the necessity of immediate specialist treatment, in 1000 patients with a pattern of complaints X

a. Original situation

| | Specialist treatment | | Total |
	Necessary	Not necessary	
Referred immediately	90	90	180
Not referred (or not immediately)	10	810	820
Total	100	900	1000

Pre-test probability of disease requiring specialist treatment = 100/1000 = 10%.
Sensitivity of referral = 90/100 = 90%.
Specificity of referral = 810/900 = 90%.
Likelihood ratio of referral = 90%/(100% – 90%) = 9.
Predictive value of referral = 90/180 = 50%.

b. Situation after halving the number of false-negatives

| | Specialist treatment | | Total |
	Necessary	Not necessary	
Referred immediately	95	495	590
Not referred (or not immediately)	5	405	410
Total	100	900	1000

Sensitivity of referral = 95/100 = 95%.
Specificity of referral = 405/900 = 45%.
Likelihood ratio of referral = 95%/(100% – 45%) = 1.7.
Predictive value of referral = 95/590 = 16%.

Specialists who provide feedback and training for GPs will often urge them to reduce the number of patients who are initially missed and who reach the specialist "too late" (bottom left category). Far less attention will be paid to patients who were referred correctly and in time (top left category) and to those who turn out to have been unnecessarily referred (top right category). No attention at all goes to those who were not referred and did not need to be (bottom right category). These last two groups are of no concern to the specialist, but they highlight one of the primary tasks of the GP: preventing unnecessary referrals. Suppose that the disproportionate attention given to the bottom left group leads to a situation in which 5 of the 10 patients in this group are referred immediately. Since the symptoms do not allow these patients to be distinguished from those in the bottom right category, half of the 810 patients who originally ended up here will now also be referred immediately (Table 6.3b). The GP's sensitivity increases a bit, from 90% to 95%, but the specificity dramatically decreases from 90% to 45%! The likelihood ratio is reduced from 9 to 1.7. The predictive value of the referral has decreased from 50% to 16%. This process may continue, if one wishes, to have the five remaining persons in the bottom left category referred immediately as well. In the end, all 1000 patients will be referred immediately. In that situation, the GP's gatekeeping function has completely disappeared, and the problem of distinguishing the two categories is shifted entirely to the specialist. Apart from the extra costs, the consequences in terms of unnecessary treatment may be enormous and the diagnostic investigations required will put a great strain on the specialist. Furthermore, the specialist has one major disadvantage: he/she lacks the all-round expertise of the GP, and many diagnostic hypotheses are outside his/her scope. What if all patients with unexplained fatigue, which may indicate hypothyroidism but usually result from non-somatic problems, were immediately referred to the endocrinologist?

Clearly, general practice is a cornerstone of our health care system.[26] The training of, and evidence-based support for the equilibrist GP, who balances between the "malpractice committee category" (bottom left) and the "medicalisation category" (top right), is a sine qua non.

Checklist for evidence-based diagnostic decision-making in general practice

(1) How do you rank your diagnostic hypotheses according to (estimated) pre-test probability, severity and therapeutical consequences?

(2) Which diagnostic test(s) is (are) most useful in an early phase with a broad problem space?

(3) What is the expected diagnostic gain of testing?

    (a) Would testing induce a clinically relevant shift from pre-test to post-test probability?

        Is the pre-test probability in the "indicated range" (not too low, not too high)?

    (b) Would the result of the considered test influence diagnostic or therapeutic management?

(c) Can the test provide doctor and patient with relevant prognostic information?

(4) Is specific evidence available on pre-test probabilities and on the discriminative power of the considered test(s) (sensitivity, specificity, likelihood ratios, predictive values)? Is this evidence valid/reliable? (For example was there an independent blind comparison of the test to a "reference standard" of diagnosis?; was the test applied to an appropriate broad spectrum of patients?; was the reference standard applied regardless of the result of test being assessed?). Which test has the highest discriminative power for testing the considered diagnostic hypotheses? Does the available evidence apply to a GP setting similar to yours?

(5) Has the trade-off profile for testing and not testing (for each considered test) been assessed?

(6) Do more tests (for example clustered tests) yield more correct and relevant information than one test?

(7) Can more evidence-based testing be promoted, either:
   (a) Individually, for example by (mutual) feedback or audit?
   (b) Generally, for example by primary care based research on the diagnostic value of diagnostic testing?

References

1 Knottnerus JA. Interpretation of diagnostic data, an unexplored field in general practice. *J R Coll Gen Pract* 1985;35:270–4.
2 Dombal FT de. Transporting databanks of medical information from one location to another. *Effective Health Care* 1983;1:155–62.
3 Williamson HA. Lymphadenopathy in a family practice: a descriptive study of 249 cases. *J Fam Pract* 1985;20:449–52.
4 Knottnerus JA, Leffers P. The influence of referral patterns on the characteristics of diagnostic tests. *J Clin Epidemiol* 1992;45:1143–54.
5 Ellenberg JH, Nelson KB. Sample selection and the natural history of disease: studies of febrile seizures. *JAMA* 1980;243:1337–40.
6 Bentveldsen FM, Schröder FH. Modalities available for screening for prostate cancer. *Eur J Cancer* 1993;29a:804–11.
7 Sheenan M, Haytorn P. Predictive values of various liver function tests with respect to the diagnosis of liver disease. *Clin Biochem* 1979;12:262–3.
8 Sackett DL, Haynes RB, Guyatt GH, Tugwell P. *Clinical epidemiology: a basic science for clinical medicine*, 2nd edn. Toronto: Little, Brown and Co., 1991.
9 Pryor DB, Shaw L, McCants CB, *et al.* Value of the history and physical in identifying patients at increased risk for coronary artery disease. *Ann Intern Med* 1993;118:81–90.
10 Panzer RJ, Black ER, Griner PF (eds). *Diagnostic strategies for common medical problems*. Philadelphia: American College of Physicians, 1991.
11 Sox HC Jr (ed). *Common diagnostic tests. Use and interpretation*, 2nd edn. Philadelphia: American College of Physicians, 1990.
12 Brooks SC, Potter BT, Rainey JB. Inversion injuries of the ankle: clinical assessment and radiographic review. *BMJ* 1981;282:607–8.

13 *Morbidity figures from general practice*. Department of General Practice. Nijmegen University, 1985.

14 Stiell IG, Greenberg GH, McKnight RD, Nair RC, McDowell I, Worthington JR. A study to develop clinical decision rules for use of radiography in acute ankle injuries. *Ann Emerg Med* 1992;**21**:384–90.

15 Stiell I, Wells G, Laupacis A, Brison R, *et al*. Multicentre trial to introduce the Ottawa ankle rules for use of radiography in acute ankle injuries. *BMJ* 1995;**311**:594–7.

16 Kroenke K, Hanley JF, Copley JB, *et al*. Improving house staff ordering of three common laboratory tests. Reduction in test ordering need not result in underutilization. *Med Care* 1987;**25**:928–35.

17 Winkens RAG, Grol RPTM, Beusmans GHMI, Kester ADM, Knottnerus JA, Pop P. Does a reduction in general practitioners' use of diagnostic tests lead to more hospital referrals? *Br J Gen Pract* 1995;**45**:289–92.

18 Knottnerus JA. Medical decision making by general practitioners and specialists. *Fam Pract* 1991;**8**:305–7.

19 Knottnerus JA, Knipschild PG, van Wersch JWJ, Sijstermans AHJ. Unexplained fatigue and haemoglobin concentration; a study in general practice patients. *Can Fam Phys* 1986;**32**:1601–4.

20 Dinant GJ, Knottnerus JA, van Wersch JW. Discriminating ability of the erythrocyte sedimentation rate: a prospective study in general practice. *Br J Gen Pract* 1991;**41**:365–70.

21 Baselier PJAM. *Urinary tract infections in general practice*. Thesis, Department of General Practice, University of Nijmegen, 1983.

22 Winkens RAG, Leffers P, Trienekens TAM, Stobberingh EE. The validity of urine examination for urinary tract infections in daily practice. *Fam Pract* 1995;**12**:290–3.

23 Winkens RAG, Pop P, Bugter AMA, *et al*. Randomised controlled trial of routine individual feedback to improve rationality and reduce numbers of test requests. *Lancet* 1995;**345**:498–502.

24 Tierney WM, Miller ME, McDonald CJ. The effect on test ordering of informing physicians of the charges for outpatient diagnostic tests. *New Engl J Med* 1990;**322**:1499–504.

25 Tierney WM, McDonald CJ, Hui SL, Martin DK. Computer predictions of abnormal test results; effects on outpatient testing. *JAMA* 1988;**259**:1194–8.

26 Starfield B. Is primary care essential? *Lancet* 1994;**344**:1129–33.

7: How to assess the effectiveness of applying the evidence

RICHARD BAKER AND RICHARD GROL

Why assess effectiveness?

Implementing change in performance is not easy. All too often, strategies used to bring about change turn out to be less effective than expected, and sometimes they have no effect whatsoever. This problem should not be surprising when it is remembered that a wide range of factors can influence the performance of professionals, the success of implementation and thus the outcomes of care. These include the nature of the change itself, characteristics of the setting, attributes of health professionals who are being asked to change their performance and the types of patients concerned.[1,2] However, it follows that plans to modify our practice should be accompanied by assessment to ensure that change has taken place. It is only by the collection of objective data on actual practice and outcomes of care that the fact of change can be confirmed.

Many practical methods are available for assessing the effectiveness of attempts to apply the evidence; these are outlined in this chapter and illustrated by examples. Other chapters in this book have made clear that by applying a few practical principles it is possible to locate and appraise research evidence and to select methods of implementation that are most likely to lead to that evidence being followed. It is important that the same systematic approach is used in assessing adherence to the evidence. After going to the trouble of finding and implementing evidence it would be inappropriate to use sloppy methods of assessment. Methods are available that do not require the collection of large amounts of data or complex analyses, but just as it is important to take a critical view of research, it is also necessary to critically appraise plans for assessment.

The most useful assessments are those that are practical to apply but also provide valid information about the most relevant aspects of care in a form that is easy to understand. There are several methods of assessing the effectiveness of the application of evidence – i.e. whether the evidence has been applied and whether its application has actually had an effect on outcome – that can possess these attributes when used appropriately, and each method has features suited to particular circumstances. In general, the methods can be divided into those that can be used by primary care practitioners and their teams, and those that may be used by other organisations that are assisting practitioners to implement change. Methods that can be used by practitioners themselves will be discussed first.

Assessment by primary care practitioners

Audit

Audit consists of a series of steps (Box 7.1) beginning with the specification of appropriate care, usually in the form of statements called review criteria – "systematically developed statements that can be used to assess the appropriateness of specific health care decisions, services and outcomes".[3] Data collection follows, and any discrepancies in performance are addressed by the use of selected implementation strategies. After a suitable period data are collected once again to check that the desired improvements have actually taken place.

Box 7.1 The stages of audit

1 Specification of criteria for appropriate care
2 Collection of data about performance
3 Comparison of performance with criteria
4 Implementation of change
5 Collection of data to check that changes have occurred

Box 7.2 shows an example of an audit undertaken by an individual practitioner. An issue was identified from a recent guideline, the group of patients concerned was easily identified and a reminder used to ensure that care would be reviewed with each patient. This audit was simple and required almost no planning. More organisation is needed if the topic is more complex, or if more members of the practice are involved.

Box 7.3 shows an example of an audit undertaken by a team concerned about a non-clinical issue. The team had to agree that the issue of the availability of routine non-urgent appointments was one that deserved attention. They also had to reach agreement on the level of performance they wished to achieve, then plan and undertake data collection, consider the results, and design and introduce a new appointment system. The successful co-ordination of these activities placed demands on practice management as several of the steps involved negotiation and the delegation of tasks such as data analysis. Whilst this team might have saved themselves some work by reducing the period over which they collected data, they were successful in improving the availability of appointments.

Box 7.2   Use of theophylline in asthma

Following the publication of guidelines for the management of asthma in adults,[4] Dr A noted the statement that theophylline might have a role in patients whose asthma was not controlled with high dose inhaled steroids, but even then alternative treatment might have fewer side-effects. He decided it was time to review his prescribing of theophylline and used the practice computer to produce a list of all his asthmatic patients and their recent medication. He found 86 patients, three of whom were taking theophylline. He was reassured that his use of theophylline was limited, but made an entry in the records of each of these patients to remind him to review their medication when the patient next attended. Ultimately, he was able to persuade two of these patients to discontinue theophylline, and after 6 months the prescribing data were checked again to confirm that these changes had persisted.

Box 7.3   Delays for routine appointments

Evidence indicates that patients in the UK become increasingly dissatisfied if there are delays for routine appointments, particularly if they have to wait longer than three days.[5-7] A primary care team agreed that patients ought to be able to see the doctor of their choice within three working days, but to take into account the problems that would arise because of holidays and other reasons for doctors' absences, they set a target of 80% for the proportion of occasions on which they thought the 3-day limit should be achieved. Over a 6-month period, at the same time each day the number of days before the next routine appointment was counted for each practitioner. The team failed to meet their target, with the 3-day limit being met on only 58% of occasions. As a result, they redesigned the appointment system and a later data collection showed that performance had improved, with compliance with the 3-day limit on 81% of occasions.

Assessing effectiveness in the local practitioner group: peer review

A particularly good tool for assessing the use of research evidence in the many countries that have large numbers of single-handed and small practices is the practitioner group. The group includes local general practitioners and meets regularly to review each other's performance and implement necessary changes in practice.[8] In these groups, indicators can be selected, data collected and exchanged and arrangements for improving care discussed and planned.

Usually this type of quality improvement is undertaken by a group or team of five to ten practitioners over an extended period. A variety of subjects, interventions and methods are used in a planned and structured way. The process may include audit, consensus development (developing agreement on criteria and targets for improvement), performance review (observation in practice by one or more colleagues), industrial quality circles (identifying and solving concrete problems in care provision) and small group education on new guidelines or evidence.

Collaboration with respected peers, making use of their evaluations and support, is central to this approach. Ideally, the different activities are integrated as part of a long term process of continuous quality improvement. This approach is a common quality improvement method in primary care in many European countries (the Netherlands, Germany, Switzerland, Ireland, Sweden and others).[9] In the Netherlands, specific educational programmes have been developed to introduce national clinical guidelines into local peer review groups. Data collection sheets with key indicators derived from the guidelines have been developed for use in the local groups. Participants collect data on their management of conditions covered by the guidelines, for example low back pain, asthma or diabetes. They can then exchange and compare their results and arrange to make the necessary changes in their performance.

Assessment by other staff or organisations

Although peer review often involves practitioners from different practices, this section is concerned with assessment undertaken or mediated by individuals or organisations other than the practitioners themselves. Health authorities, primary care groups, funders, professional associations or colleges, or agencies acting on behalf of primary care teams may take the lead in this process. External practice assessment is also sometimes undertaken to monitor contracts, allocate resources or determine the need for other types of management intervention. However, this type of performance monitoring will not be considered in this chapter.

One example of cooperation between practices through an intermediate organisation to assess care is provided by the many clinical audit projects undertaken in the UK clinical governance programme.[10] A local group is funded by the health authority to organise such projects, and teams are invited to take part. Provided the criteria on which these audits are based are related to research evidence, information can be provided to the participating teams to show how they compare with their colleagues. An example is discussed in Box 7.4.

In some Scandinavian countries, a similar method for enabling practitioners to collect information about aspects of performance for comparison with others has been established. Large numbers of practitioners take part, and in addition to the data collection, training courses are organised to implement the guidelines developed for each topic.[12] To ensure standard data collection, a registration form is developed for prospective completion by the participating practitioners immediately after each consultation with a patient with the topic in question (Figure 7.1). Another example of a similar approach is shown in Box 7.5.

In some countries, there are programmes for the development and implementation of guidelines which contain evidence-based

---

Box 7.4 An audit of the management of long-term benzodiazepine users in 18 general practices

The local group of health professionals decided to undertake an audit of the management of patients taking benzodiazepines (anxiolytics and hypnotics) long term, defined as four weeks or longer. Criteria were developed following a literature review, and data were collected from the records of random samples of patients in the 18 practices that agreed to take part. On average, patients had been taking their medication for 10 years, and there were wide gaps between the elements of management recommended in the literature and that indicated by the records. Following feedback to each practice of their performance in comparison with the other anonymous practices, significant improvements in care took place, including the withdrawal of a proportion of patients from their medication.[11]

---

recommendations. In the Netherlands, guidelines are developed in a rigorous step-wise process that takes up to one and a half years per guideline.[13] To evaluate the use of these guidelines in practice, various methods are used – self-recording (Box 7.6), chart audit, observation, computerised monitoring.

Box 7.5 Evaluation of adherence to the evidence: national information network for primary health care

A national network for collecting aggregated and representative data from primary health care has been set up by two professional organisations in the Netherlands, the NIVEL Institute and the Centre for Quality of Care Research (WOK). Over 100 practices, representative of the national population of practices, are using computerised information and recording systems to continuously record and periodically collect information on diagnoses, referrals, prescriptions, test ordering, preventive procedures and adherence to national practice guidelines. Practices receive feedback that they can use in their quality improvement activities.[13]

How to assess effectiveness of applying evidence: basic principles

An essential requirement for assessing the effectiveness of applying the evidence is good quality data about actual performance. These data must be accurate and genuinely represent performance if the findings are to be used as the starting point for implementation of improvements in care. Unfortunately, mistakes in collecting data are common, but by following a few simple rules these can usually be avoided (Box 7.7).

It is important to begin by developing clear and explicit review criteria. These should be expressed in terms that specify exactly what information should be sought, and research evidence should be the starting point for their development, each criterion being justified by the strength of the

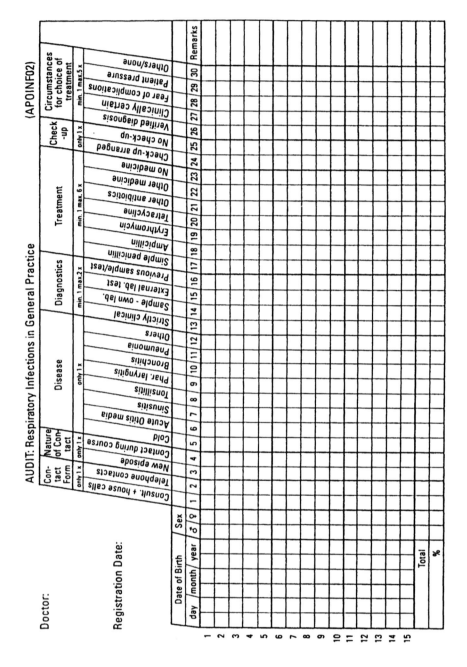

Fig 7.1 A registration form for respiratory infections in general practice. Reproduced with permission from Munck.[12]

Box 7.6 Assessing adherence to clinical practice guidelines in local general practitioner groups

To evaluate the use of research evidence, summarised in national evidence based guidelines for general practice in the Netherlands,[13,14] 65 general practitioners recorded their performance immediately after consultation for 30 different guidelines on specially designed recording sheets containing a selection of indicators for use of the guidelines and evidence. The reliability of recording was checked by comparison with observation by a trained observer in a sample of consultations. A total of 3600 consultations were assessed in this manner, and about 20 000 different actions and decisions could be compared with recommendations in the guidelines. On average, almost 70% of the recommendations were followed in practice. There were, however, large differences between different guidelines (range 40–90%) and between individual practitioners (range <50 to >80%), in adherence to the guidelines.[13]

---

evidence and the impact on outcome.[15] To check that the criteria are appropriately worded and feasible to use, they can be tested in a pilot involving the collection of data about the care of a small number of patients.

Box 7.7 Requirements for collecting data to assess care

1 Evidence based criteria or indicators
2 Complete and accurate list of patients
3 Representative samples
4 Reliable data extraction
5 Meaningful data analysis

Once a satisfactory set of criteria has been selected, the patients whose care is to be assessed must be identified. This may be done retrospectively or prospectively, via a range of sources whose pros and cons, with respect to the relevance and validity of the data derived from them, are discussed in more detail below. In prospective data collection, the patients included are usually restricted to those who consult within a predefined period of time or until a predetermined number of patients have been seen. A complete and accurate list of patients is essential to prevent mistaken conclusions being drawn, as the care of patients on the list may differ from those who are not. It is important to ensure that every eligible patient is included, as, for example, the doctors may be tempted to exclude those who present with more difficult clinical problems. Furthermore, different types of patients may consult at different times of the year, for example patients with certain respiratory infections may consult in parallel with the seasonal variation in prevalence of the organism responsible.

Once a list of patients has been compiled, it may be necessary to select a sample if the total numbers involved are substantial. Samples must be representative and also sufficiently large to ensure confidence in the findings. Random sampling can usually be undertaken without great difficulty. A number is assigned to each patient, and a table of random numbers consulted to indicate which ones to include.[16] Pocket calculators can also generate random numbers. The calculation of sample size can appear difficult, but this need not be the case. Simple advice is available,[16,17] and an easy to use software program which can calculate sample sizes is widely available (EPI INFO).

However, when patient numbers are scarce, for example in the assessment of issues related to uncommon conditions such as meningitis, it may not be possible to recruit enough patients to allow for meaningful and valid data analysis. In this situation, "significant event audit", as discussed later, may be the only practical method of assessment of the effectiveness of the application of evidence.

Each data source has advantages and disadvantages. The ideal source is practical to use and provides data that are relevant and valid.

Practicality is the first point to consider. It is essential, but it should not overrule the need for relevance and validity. If this is allowed to happen, assessment becomes restricted to those aspects of care that are easily measured. By using samples of patients from a combination of sources, it is often possible to collect data that are relevant and valid, but also convenient and cheap to obtain.

Relevance is the next point to consider. The data source must relate to the criteria. For example, clinical records would be unlikely to contain relevant information about the extent to which patients are involved in decisions. Video, audiotape or a patient questionnaire would be more likely to provide relevant material.

Validity should be considered next. Many factors can influence validity, and each source and method of data collection has its own potential problems. The ability of patients to recall aspects of their consultations may reduce the validity of questionnaires, encounter sheets may prompt practitioners and therefore fail to reflect usual performance, and paper or computer recording systems are often incomplete. In a comparison of clinical records and audiotapes of consultations, general practitioners recorded information about smoking advice on only 25% of occasions that it was given.[18] Depending on the review criteria, it may be necessary to use a combination of data sources to ensure validity.

In order to obtain valid data it is important to ensure that data collection from clinical records occurs in a reproducible manner. Different people may interpret the contents of records in different ways, and apparent differences in the quality of care provided by two practices are due solely to the way in which items in records were interpreted. Therefore, explicit data extraction rules are needed. In research studies, checks of data collection reliability are undertaken, and sometimes these can be necessary in assessments of other areas of performance. Using a small random sample of records, data are independently extracted by two data collectors and their findings compared. Ideally they should be in full agreement, and the percentage agreement can be assessed, or a measure of reliability such as kappa can be calculated.[16]

Although on many occasions clinical records will be the source of data, there are alternatives such as encounter sheets (Figure 7.1) or computer-held data (Box 7.5). Some aspects of care may initially appear more difficult to measure, but the combination of careful planning and methods of data collection such as patient questionnaires, qualitative interviews, or observation by video or audiotape, can often provide revealing and meaningful data provided explicit review criteria are identified beforehand.

To draw conclusions about the effectiveness of applying the evidence, information about performance is compared to the recommendations from research evidence. The data are usually expressed as "proportions", that is, the proportion of patients whose care is in compliance with the evidence. The use of complex statistical tests is generally unnecessary, but if patient samples have been used it is helpful to employ a measure which takes into account the possibility of lack of precision. The confidence interval defines the range of values that has a particular probability of containing the population's true proportion. Put simply, a 95% confidence interval for a sample indicates that there is a 95% chance that the interval includes the true population proportion whose care complies with the evidence. For most types of data collected to assess the effectiveness of applying the evidence, the calculation of confidence intervals is relatively straightforward.[19] An example is shown in Box 7.8. A two sample confidence interval calculation is used to compare the data from two data collections, for example the first and second in an audit by one team, or the findings from a single data collection in two different teams.[20]

Should we assess process or outcome?

In assessing the application of evidence in daily practice, effectiveness can be viewed in one of two ways. From one perspective, effectiveness can be interpreted as meaning the degree of success of attempts to ensure the compliance of practitioners with the evidence. Assessment of effectiveness would then consist of the collection of data about the performance of the practitioners involved and direct comparison of the findings with the recommendations arising from the evidence. This is sometimes referred to as assessment of the *process* of care.

An alternative view of effectiveness is that care provided by practitioners leads to the outcomes that research has shown can be achieved if the evidence is applied correctly. Assessment would then consist of the collection of information about the *outcome* of care.

Box 7.8   Calculating confidence intervals in an audit

One primary care team taking part in the audit of benzodiazepine prescribing (Box 7.4) was particularly interested in whether patients had been offered help with withdrawal. They chose, as a target, 60% of patients having a record in their notes of being offered help. In the first data collection, only 44% of the sampled patients had such a record. They calculated the 95% confidence interval for this result, following Gardner and Altman,[20] as follows:

$$\left[p \pm 1.96\sqrt{\frac{p(1-p)}{n}} \right]$$

where p = the proportion being offered withdrawal (44%), and n the sample size (134 patients). Thus, the 95% confidence interval was 44% plus or minus 8.4% (35.6%–52.4%). The target of 60% was outside the confidence intervals, indicating that they had indeed failed to reach their target.

If outcomes prove poorer than expected, one explanation might be that the practitioners had not fully complied with the evidence, but another might be that the patients they were treating were more unwell than those included in the research studies and consequently suffered a poorer outcome. Thus, assessment of outcome can be an indirect way of assessing the practitioners' use of evidence. If our aim is to assess the quality of care, the use of outcome assessment would be reasonable, but if the aim is more narrowly concerned with the degree to which actual care is in compliance with evidence, direct assessment of process is necessary. This chapter is concerned with assessing the extent to which care is in accordance with evidence and therefore assessment of process has been emphasised, although for some conditions outcome measurement may be used. Examples include investigation of the proportion of patients with chronic obstructive pulmonary disease (COPD) who discontinue smoking after receiving advice and support, or the proportion of hypertensive patients whose blood pressure is controlled within a target range (Box 7.9).

Managing assessment of effectiveness

Primary care practitioners provide care to patients with almost all types of illness, and at the same time they have to manage systems such as appointments, recall schemes and screening services in a way that complies with the wishes and needs of their patients. The identification and implementation of evidence-based practice are additional activities which also require time and energy, and to expect assessment to be routinely undertaken for every new item of research evidence is unrealistic. If a primary care team is to respond systematically to recommendations arising from new evidence, mechanisms are needed for identifying these

---

Box 7.9 Asthma and COPD monitoring[24]

As part of a project on the implementation of clinical guidelines for asthma and COPD care, the participating practitioners continuously monitor specific information about their patients. A selection of indicators derived from the guideline, is used including: decline in lung function (peak flow measurement, spirometry), patients' smoking habits, patients' compliance with follow up appointments and use of anti-inflammatory medication in patients needing more than two daily doses of bronchodilator. This information provides immediate feedback to the general practitioner on the fulfilment of some of the aims of the guideline in individual patients.

---

recommendations and for deciding which are most important. This implies the need for active management of the introduction of evidence-based medicine, with agreed structures and policies to enable this to take place.[21,22] The precise nature of these arrangements will vary according to the team and the characteristics of health care systems in different countries, but the principle is transferable: the effective introduction of evidence-based practice, rather than merely the introduction of a few aspects of care which are evidence-based, is a process that requires effective management. Some of the factors that need to be taken into account are shown in Box 7.10. In addition to audit and peer review, information from significant events and continuous systematic monitoring can play an important role in this regard, as already discussed.

Significant event audit

The systematic use of isolated episodes to detect possible deficiencies in care can be a useful component of any plan to introduce evidence-based care. All practitioners are curious about the consequences of their decisions in the management of patients. Reflection is an inherent component of clinical practice, and often arises from the failure of some patients to progress as expected, the practitioner then considering whether an alternative treatment or a different choice of words in the consultation would have been better. Omissions in previous episodes of care may be triggers for reflection, for example the case of a 70-year-old man whose rectal bleeding was at first thought to be due to his long-standing haemorrhoids, who returns after a month and is found to have a rectal mass, or a middle aged woman who presents with depression with no discernable precipitants, until her husband tells you that their daughter left home 6 months ago and they have not heard from her since. Why were you unable to get the patient to tell you this herself? Events like these are not uncommon in primary care and provide anecdotes for discussion with colleagues and opportunities for learning.

Having decided to comply with a new piece of research evidence, the practitioner is likely to take note of, and reflect upon his or her own

---

Box 7.10   Some factors to be taken into account by practice management in managing procedures to assess the effectiveness of applying the evidence

Setting priorities:
National policies and guidelines
Priorities of the local health authority
Local patients' needs due to factors such as level of deprivation, disease incidence, age of population
Less obvious issues, e.g. practitioner–patient relationships

Practice resources:
Level of teamwork
Computer systems
Availability of evidence, e.g. practice library, Medline access, Cochrane library on CD-ROM
Existing quality assurance mechanisms
Staff with time and skill to take on particular role, e.g. data collection, appraisal of guidelines, etc.
Information about significant events

Local resources:
Clinical library
Expertise in postgraduate or university departments of general practice
Training for general practitioners and practice staff in audit or monitoring methods
Peer review groups

---

performance. The advantages of this type of assessment are that it does not require additional resources or detailed preparation, can be used even with uncommon conditions and it provides live information about specific patients. However, there are disadvantages because it is not systematic and may only include selected types of patients, such as those who consult frequently.

Despite these difficulties it can be useful in two circumstances. Firstly, if the clinical condition is one with a low incidence there may be no other practical method of assessment: for example, in the management of acute illness in the community such as meningitis, myocardial infarction or status epilepticus, only analysis of isolated events is possible. Secondly, individual episodes can be used as markers to indicate that more detailed assessment is needed to check whether there is a more general problem. When used systematically, this method is referred to as "significant event audit",[23] in which members of the team record such episodes so that they may be discussed later and decisions made about how to respond to them. A further advantage of this method is that it helps to encourage an attitude of self-monitoring (Box 7.11).

Box 7.11   The diagnosis of colorectal cancer

Stimulated by a delay in the diagnosis of rectal cancer in one patient, a practitioner decided to investigate the time it had taken her to make this diagnosis in other patients. This type of investigation is called "delay pattern analysis". She identified the last five patients who had been found to have colorectal cancer from the practice computer. For two, the diagnosis had been made at the first consultation; the delay for the others had been 4, 8 and 9 weeks. She decided to refresh her skills in the use of sigmoidoscopy.

Systematic monitoring

Another method of collecting data to assess the effectiveness of applying the evidence is "systematic monitoring", which is becoming more common and practical with the wide use of computerised information systems. Specific data are continuously collected, using selected relevant indicators derived from the evidence. This is a particularly useful method for monitoring the quality of care for chronic diseases (eg diabetes or asthma).

In the project outlined in Box 7.9,[24] involving all patients with asthma and chronic obstructive pulmonary disease (COPD) in 12 practices, practitioners are continuously monitoring computerised data. The data are used to evaluate whether key targets of the national guidelines for asthma and COPD management are being achieved. For the practitioners, the data provide immediate feedback on individual patients, which can be used to adapt care provision.

Until recently, such monitoring has been inhibited by the problem of extracting data from the wide variety of computer systems used by general practitioners. However, methods of extracting data from different systems to enable comparison are becoming available. As this work progresses, it is becoming clear that different primary care teams use their computer systems in different ways, and some are more sophisticated users than others. In order to ensure comparable data, practices will have to agree to record clinical information in a uniform rather than idiosyncratic way, and all will have to become proficient computer users.

Conclusions

The assumption that we will automatically comply with the recommendations of guidelines or new research evidence is naive. However, there is a great deal that we can do both individually and as members of health care teams to assess how well we are applying the evidence. We should then use the findings to guide the application of systematic steps to close the gap between actual performance and research evidence. In this chapter a variety of practical methods have been described which can be used to check performance, and the main principles relating to their use have been discussed.

Firstly, the data to be collected should be based on the evidence. Secondly, although the choice of method of data collection will be influenced by the type and number of practitioners or practices involved, it is important to select the one that is the most practical, relevant and valid. Thirdly, attention should be paid to the rigour of data collection methods including identification of all involved patients, appropriateness of samples and the use of confidence intervals if samples are used, and the reliability of data extraction. It is wise to make use of external sources of support such as peer review groups or other local resources. Finally, the introduction of evidence-based practice and its assessment is more likely to be accomplished when managed systematically. Teams should begin to regard the implementation of evidence as one task for practice management, rather than leave it to the vagaries of individual professional habits.

References

1 Davis DA, Thomson MA, Oxman AD, Haynes RB. Changing physician performance. A systematic review of the effect of continuing medical education strategies. *JAMA* 1995;**274**:700–5.
2 Wensing M, Grol R. Single and combined strategies for implementing changes in primary care: a literature review. *Int J Quality Health Care* 1994;**6**:115–32.
3 Institute of Medicine. *Guidelines for clinical practice. From development to use.* Washington, DC: National Academy Press, 1992.
4 British Thoracic Society. Guidelines on the management of asthma. *Thorax* 1993;**48**(supplement): S1–S24.
5 Cartwright A, Anderson R. *General practice revisited.* London: Tavistock, 1981.
6 Allen D, Leavey R, Marks B. Survey of patients' satisfaction with access to general practitioners. *J Roy Coll Gen Pract* 1988;**38**:163–5.
7 Beckham R. Getting to see your GP. *Which?* 1993; March:11–14.
8 Grol R, Lawrence M. *Quality improvement by peer review.* Oxford: Oxford University Press, 1995.
9 Grol R. Quality improvement by peer review in primary care: a practical guide. *Quality Health Care* 1994;**3**:147–52.
10 Baker R, Lakhani M, Fraser RC, Cheater F. A model for clinical governance in primary care groups. *BMJ* 1999;**318**:779–83.
11 Baker R, Farooqi A, Tait C, Walsh S. A randomised controlled trial of reminders to enhance the impact of audit on management of benzodiazepine users in general practice. *Quality Health Care* 1997;**6**:14–18.
12 Munck A. Audit project Odense (APO) – a Scandinavian audit centre for general practice. *Audit Trends* 1995;**3**:18–21.
13 Grol R, Thomas S, Roberts R. Development and implementation of guidelines for family practice: lessons from the Netherlands. *J Fam Pract* 1995;**40**:435–9.
14 Grol R. Development of guidelines for general practice care. *Br J Gen Pract* 1993;**43**:146–51.
15 Baker R, Fraser RC. Development of review criteria: linking guidelines and assessment of quality. *BMJ* 1995;**311**:370–3.
16 Altman DG. *Practical statistics for medical research.* London: Chapman & Hall, 1991.
17 Mant D, Yudkin P. Collecting and analysing data. In: Lawrence M, Schofield T, eds. *Medical audit in primary health care.* Oxford: Oxford University Press, 1993, pp 56–75.

18 Wilson A, McDonald P. Comparison of patient questionnaire, medical record and audio tape in assessment of health promotion in general practice consultation. *BMJ* 1994;**209**:1483–5.
19 Evidence Based Care Resource Group. Evidence based care: 3 Measuring performance: how are we managing this problem? *Can Med Assoc J* 1994;**150**:1575–9.
20 Gardner MJ, Altman DG. *Statistics with confidence – confidence intervals and statistical guidelines*. London: BMJ Publishing Group, 1989.
21 Irvine D, Irvine S. *The practice of quality*. Oxford: Radcliffe Medical Press, 1996.
22 Hearnshaw HM, Baker RH, Robertson N. Multidisciplinary audit in primary health care teams: facilitation by audit support staff. *Quality Health Care* 1994;**3**:164–8.
23 Pringle M, Bradley CP, Carmichael CM, Wallis H, Moore A. *Significant event auditing. A study of the feasibility and potential of case-based auditing in primary medical care*. Occasional paper 70. London: Royal College of General Practitioners, 1995.
24 Centre for Quality of Care Research. *Research programme and results*. Nijmegen: WOK, 1997.

Part 2 – Strategies to develop a culture of evidence-based health care in primary care

8: An overview of strategies to promote implementation of evidence-based health care

ANDREW D OXMAN AND SIGNE FLOTTORP

Introduction

Evidence is essential but not sufficient for evidence-based practice. At least three types of information and three types of judgements are needed for well-informed decisions (Figure 8.1). First, clinical judgement is needed to identify and diagnose health problems, to learn which health outcomes are important to the patient and to identify which preventive, diagnostic, treatment, or rehabilitation options should be considered. Information for this must be collected from the patient (through history taking, physical examination and diagnostic tests). Second, to estimate the effects of different options on health outcomes, judgements must be made about effectiveness and adverse effects. This information comes from comparative studies, particularly systematic reviews of reliable evidence.[1] It is also

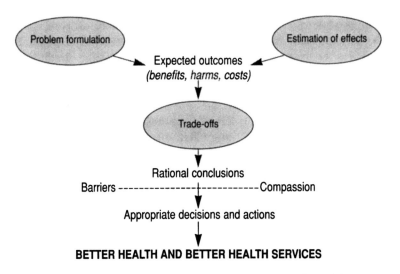

Fig 8.1 Types of information and judgements in implementing evidence.

important to consider the applicability of comparative studies, diagnostic accuracy and prognostic factors.[2]

These first two types of judgements and information taken together provide estimates of the expected outcomes associated with the options that are considered. It is then necessary to make judgements about trade-offs between the expected benefits, harms and costs. Sometimes formal economic or decision analysis is used to clarify the trade-offs. Whether this is done formally or informally, information is needed about the "value" or desirability of the outcomes from the perspective of those who are affected, most importantly the patient. In addition, ethical and cultural values must be taken into account. For example, for obstetric technologies it is frequently necessary to find a balance between autonomy (a woman's right to make her own choices) and beneficence (towards both the unborn child and the mother).

These three types of judgements and information taken together can provide the basis for rational conclusions about how to manage a health problem. For rational conclusions to be translated into effective practice, at least two other factors must be considered. Barriers to implementing appropriate actions must be identified and addressed[3] and compassion must be considered. Health care that is compassionate but not rational is likely to be inefficient at best, and may do more harm than good. On the other hand, health care that is rational without being compassionate may also do more harm than good. Empathy and compassion are necessary in establishing a good relationship between providers and recipients of care and to ensure that patients' needs and anxieties are recognised and addressed. Health care based on evidence but without compassion may harm patients and is likely to be less efficient than care that is based on both evidence and empathy (Box 8.1).

Although patients want effective care and health care providers want to provide this, gaps are frequently found between evidence-based decisions and what is done in practice. There are a variety of reasons for these gaps. Consequently, a variety of strategies may be needed to reduce them. For example, clinicians may not have the information they need and may not even be aware of this,[3] they may feel pressured by patients to refer them unnecessarily,[4] may order unnecessary diagnostic tests because of concern about liability,[5] or may feel compelled to practise according to local standards even when these are not evidence-based.[6]

In this chapter we present an overview of how to identify barriers to evidence-based practice, how to tailor implementation strategies to address identified barriers, and how to assess whether implementation strategies do what they are intended to do. We conclude by discussing the need for collaboration.

Box 8.1 Types of information and judgements in implementing evidence: preventive hormone therapy (PHT) for postmenopausal women

Example (PHT)

Problem formulation
↓

Information is needed from the patient about her age, menopause, risk factors for osteoporosis, coronary heart disease, endometrial cancer, breast cancer. Clinical judgement must be used in deciding when and how to collect this information, among other things in relation to the patient's expectations and resources. The availability of other options (for example, alendronate) and local circumstances must also be considered (for example, whether PHT and other options are covered or must be paid for out of pocket), as well as cultural and personal attitudes (for example, regarding taking medications or vaginal bleeding).

Estimation of effects
↓

Information is needed, preferably from systematic reviews, about the effects of PHT on osteoporotic fractures, coronary heart disease, life expectancy, endometrial cancer, breast cancer, side-effects, and vaginal bleeding. Judgement is required to assess the validity and applicability of this evidence.

Expected outcomes
↓

The two types of information and judgements above provide a basis for estimating the expected benefits, harms, and costs of PHT compared with no PHT or compared with other options.

Trade-offs
↓

Although societal values should be used in deciding whether or not PHT should be covered by health insurance, individual women vary in the relative value they attach to the effects of PHT, such as vaginal bleeding, and in their attitudes towards uncertainty (for example, about a possible increased risk of breast cancer). Individual rather than societal values should be used for individual patient decisions (within the economic and ethical constraints of the community).

Rational conclusions
↓

Based on the above information and judgements, a rational conclusion can be reached about whether or not to recommend or initiate PHT.

Barriers

Barriers to implementing rational decisions regarding PHT might exist for both the patient and the clinician, including inadequate time to help a patient reach an appropriate personal decision, lack of health insurance coverage, misperceptions of the risk of liability from either recommending or not recommending PHT, unrealistic patient expectations, opinions of the clinician or woman that are not consistent with the evidence and the clinician's attitudes towards prevention.

+
Compassion

⇩

A patient might, for example, have an extreme fear of breast cancer. Compassion is necessary to recognise and address this fear.

Appropriate decisions and actions

In the case of PHT, appropriate decisions and actions are likely to vary from woman to woman, even among women with the same risk factors in the same setting. Thus, while evidence is essential to reach an appropriate decision, it is clearly not sufficient either to make a decision or to ensure that the decision is acted upon.

Identifying barriers

Once a gap has been identified between what should be done in practice (based on current best evidence) and what is being done in practice, the first step towards reducing the gap is to identify the reasons why it exists. Most clinicians want to provide the best possible care for their patients. When they do not do so there is generally a good reason why. Sometimes it is simply due to a lack of knowledge. Often, however, there are other reasons. Clinical behaviour, like other behaviours (for example, physical activity, sexual behaviour, eating, smoking, drinking, adherence to medical advice) is determined by a number of factors, and the link between knowledge and behaviour is often weak. Anyone who has tried to change patient behaviour, or one's own behaviour, will recognise how difficult it is. Knowledge alone is often not sufficient for behaviour change.

Other factors that can determine clinical behaviour and act as barriers to improving clinical practice can be related for example to the practice environment, prevailing opinion and personal attitudes (Box 8.2).[7]

Practice environment

- **Financial disincentives** (lack of adequate reimbursement or a loss in income associated with the desired change in behaviour).
- **Organisational constraints** (lack of time or organisational problems in the local environment that make the desired change in behaviour difficult (for example, inaccessibility of necessary equipment or support services, or inability of the provider to access pertinent information when it is needed)).
- **Perception of liability** (perceived threat of litigation or risk of a formal complaint being filed).
- **Patient expectations** (wishes of the patient related to clinical care directly expressed to the provider or perceived by the provider).

Prevailing opinion

- **Standards of practice** (the usual practice in the setting, i.e. when this is not consistent with evidence-based recommendations).
- **Opinion leaders** (who sometimes express opinions that are not consistent with evidence-based recommendations).
- **Medical training** (which frequently becomes out of date within years of graduation but continues to influence how health professionals practise).
- **Advocacy** (for example, by pharmaceutical companies).

Box 8.2 Identifying barriers

Barriers

Practice environment	**Examples**
Financial disincentives	Reimbursement systems may promote unnecessary services, such as use of diagnostic tests and procedures, or discourage services that take time and are poorly reimbursed, such as counselling.
Organisational constraints	Burdensome paperwork or poor communication may inhibit provision of effective care. For example, effective secondary preventive measures for myocardial infarction, such as aspirin and β-blockers, may not be used because of unclear division of responsibility and poor communication between primary and secondary care providers.
Perception of liability	Physicians may order unnecessary tests, such as exercise electrocardiograms or ankle X-rays, due to their perceptions of being at risk of complaints of malpractice.
Patient expectations	Patients may expect (or physicians may perceive that they expect) antibiotics for upper respiratory infections although they are not indicated.

Prevailing opinion	
Standards of practice	Fear to practise differently than others in the community may inhibit adoption of new forms of care, such as single-dose treatment of urinary tract infections, or promote continued use of forms of care that may not be justified, such as antibiotic treatment of acute otitis media.
Opinion leaders	Local opinion leaders may encourage the use of forms of care that have not been shown to be effective, such as screening for ovarian or prostate cancer, or may discourage the use of effective forms of care, such as manipulation for low back pain.
Medical training	Clinicians may provide sub-optimal forms of care, such as continuous use of β-agonists, or may underuse effective forms of care, such as corticosteroids for asthma, because of the influence of what they learned in training on how they continue to practise.
Advocacy	Advocacy by pharmaceutical companies may promote inappropriate use of medications or unnecessary use of expensive medications, such as non-steroidal anti-inflammatory agents, broad spectrum antibiotics, or new classes of anti-hypertensive drugs.

Knowledge and attitudes	
Clinical uncertainty	Clinicians may order unnecessary tests for vague symptoms, such as diffuse pain or fatigue, "just to be sure" even though the tests are likely to result in more false than true positives, may potentially do harm, and waste resources unnecessarily.
Sense of competence	Clinicians may fail to undertake procedures or diagnostic examinations, such as proctoscopy, prescribe effective medications, such as angiotensin-converting enzyme inhibitors, or provide counselling about exercise or diet because they do not feel competent.
Compulsion to act	Clinicians may feel compelled to "do something", such as refer a patient with headache or order a CT scan, even though they are aware that there is little or no indication for doing so.
Information overload	Clinicians may fail to keep up with new developments, such as *H. pylori* eradication for dyspepsia, because they are overwhelmed with the amount of information (much of which is not relevant or valid) with which they are confronted.

Knowledge and attitudes

- **Clinical uncertainty** (discomfort with uncertainty; for example, as a potential reason for ordering unnecessary diagnostic tests).
- **Sense of competence** (provider's confidence in their own abilities; for example, as a potential reason for not performing an indicated procedure).
- **Compulsion to act** (need to "do something" even when no effective care is available).
- **Information overload** (inability to critically appraise the validity and applicability of conflicting reports).

The identification of barriers to implementing evidence-based care depends largely on qualitative methods. Critical reflection is the starting point for identifying the determinants of practice. However, reflection alone is often not adequate. Most of us have limited insight into our own motives, let alone the motives of others. Methods that can be used to assist the correct identification of barriers to implementing evidence-based guidelines in practice include semi-structured interviews, focus groups and observation. Surveys have the potential to provide quantitative data about the extent of, and variation in, barriers but they may be misleading. Direct observation may be the most valid means of identifying barriers but this is time-consuming and often not practical. Somewhat paradoxically, focus groups (facilitated group discussions) may enable more open and critical reflection than one-on-one interviews and therefore may be the best approach to identifying barriers. Most clinicians are extremely busy and finding the time to participate in group discussions about why they do what they do may, at first sight, appear like a low priority. However, such discussions can be extremely rewarding and many clinicians are, indeed, grateful for the opportunity to have an open discussion with colleagues about what they do. Hearing others admit to uncertainty or recognise problems in how they practise can stimulate more critical self-reflection and enable more openness about one's own shortcomings. Careful facilitation of such group discussions is necessary to ensure an open and receptive forum (where there are no "right" or "wrong" perceptions), obtain full participation, keep the discussion focused and use what limited time is available efficiently.

Tailoring implementation strategies to address identified barriers

After gaps between practice and evidence are recognised and the reasons for the gaps are identified, there are no magic bullets for reducing those gaps.[8] The reasons for not practising based on best current evidence vary from clinical problem to problem, and for the same clinical problem they may vary from clinician to clinician. As a result, it is necessary to tailor the implementation strategies that are used to address the specific barriers that are identified. There is a wide range of interventions available that, if used appropriately, can lead to substantial improvements in the effectiveness and efficiency of health services (Box 8.3). These include the use of well-designed educational materials and meetings, outreach visits, opinion leaders, patient-mediated interventions, audit and feedback, reminders, marketing, local consensus processes and multifaceted interventions.[9] These interventions are complex and can vary in terms of the content, source, recipient, timing and format. Interpretation of the results of evaluations of these interventions requires disentangling interactions

---

Box 8.3   Examples of interventions to change physician behaviour

Intervention	Description
Continuing medical education (CME) approaches	
Educational materials	Distribution of published or printed recommendations for clinical care, including papers, books and video or electronic material.
Conferences	Participation of health care providers in conferences, lectures and workshops.
Quality assurance (QA) approaches	
Audit and feedback	Review of the performance of health care provider over a particular period of time and provision of this information to the providers.
Reminders	Systems designed to remind clinicians or patients of information and/or desired actions. These may be manual or computerised.
Social influence approaches	
Local consensus processes	Development of local guidelines or practice protocols through participation and round table discussion.
Use of opinion leaders	Use of influential individuals who may change the attitudes and behaviours of others by personal example and influence.
Patient-mediated interventions	Interventions aimed at changing the behaviour of health care providers where information is given directly to patients, for example by direct mailing of leaflets, or patient counselling.
Targeted approaches	
Academic detailing	An educational outreach approach to providing information to practitioners, similar to activities by pharmaceutical industry sales representatives to market drugs.
Tailored interventions	Use of group discussions (focus groups), personal interviews, observation or surveys of targeted providers to identify and address barriers to changing their behaviour.

between the characteristics of the targeted professionals, the interventions, the targeted behaviours and the research design. Systematic reviews of the effects of interventions to help health care professionals improve their practice indicate that such interventions often can be effective, but are not always effective, and that the effects of even relatively complex and intensive interventions, such as outreach visits and the use of local opinion leaders, have only moderate effects of 20–50% relative improvement.[10,11]

At present, we lack sufficient evidence to provide precise guidelines for how to design an implementation strategy. Although theoretical frameworks can be helpful in guiding decisions about which types of strategies to use, there is a lack of empirical evidence to support any particular theory about how to change professional practice and there is no clear-cut basis for suggesting which specific interventions are most effective for which barriers to change. Tailoring implementation strategies requires creativity in addition to an understanding of the key barriers to change (Box 8.4). For example, Avorn and Sournerai identified three important barriers to reducing inappropriate use of vasodilators for peripheral vascular disease.[12] Doctors were reluctant to admit to patients that they had prescribed an ineffective medication because of their perceptions of the risk of litigation or how that might affect their relationship with patients. Doctors perceived that patients wanted a prescription. Doctors did not feel competent in prescribing exercise, an effective treatment. To address these barriers, doctors were offered a way of explaining to patients why the medication was being discontinued in a positive way (by explaining that it resulted from efforts to keep up to date and improve their quality of care) and they were provided with prescription pads for exercise, thus making it possible to hand patients a prescription while at the same time facilitating the provision of an appropriate prescription for exercise.

Evaluating implementation strategies

Changes in clinical behaviours are likely to be moderate, at best. Bias in evaluations of the effects of implementation strategies can be as large or larger than the effects that are being measured. Therefore, it is important to use rigorous methods to evaluate the effectiveness of implementation strategies (Box 8.5). Randomised controlled trials (RCTs) are likely to provide the best evidence of the effectiveness of implementation strategies.

When evaluating guidelines in simple (patient) randomised trials there is a danger that the treatment offered to patients in the control group will be contaminated by doctors' knowledge of the guidelines, with the result that the evaluation may underestimate the true effect.[13] In studies where doctors (or hospitals) are randomised to intervention or control groups, doctors randomised to the guidelines group may be subject to greater Hawthorne effects (the beneficial effects on performance of taking part in research)[14]

Box 8.4 Tailoring implementation strategies to address identified barriers

Examples of identified barriers

Tailored implementation strategies

Possible overuse of x rays for ankle injuries may be due to patient expectations and misperceptions of the risk of subsequent malpractice complaints.

A tailored implementation strategy to reduce unnecessary use of ankle x rays might include providing physicians with appropriate patient information regarding indications for x rays with ankle injuries and providing data and legal opinions to reassure physicians about not being at risk of malpractice complaints.

Failure to provide counselling regarding alcohol misuse may result from lack of knowledge about its effectiveness, financial or organisational disincentives that restrict the amount of time available to identify and counsel patients, and lack of a sense of competence.

A tailored implementation strategy to promote screening and counselling for alcohol misuse might include workshops with skill training using role play and case discussions, and simple strategies for providing counselling that minimise the time required of physicians (for example, by providing appropriate patient information and using other staff).

Overuse of expensive non-steroidal anti-inflammatory drugs (NSAIDS) when less expensive, equally effective, and safe alternatives are available may be due to advocacy from pharmaceutical companies, lack of knowledge or misinformation about the evidence of effectiveness and costs of the available options, and lack of awareness or feedback regarding personal practice patterns and the effects of those practice patterns on the quality of care and resource utilisation.

A tailored implementation strategy to reduce unnecessary prescribing of expensive NSAIDS might include "counter detailing" (outreach visits), provision of information about the comparative costs and effectiveness of alternative NSAIDS, provision of prescription pads for less expensive alternatives, appropriate patient information and advice about how to maximise the placebo effect when prescribing less expensive, generic alternatives (for example, by being positive), and feedback about resources saved through using less expensive, equally effective alternatives (or the opportunity costs of continuing to use unnecessarily expensive NSAIDS). Information about alternative NSAIDS, standard prescriptions, and patient information could all be computerised and provided via electronic medical record systems.

Primary care physicians may order CT scans or refer patients with headache unnecessarily due to financial disincentives that restrict them from using adequate time to take a thorough history and counsel patients, pressure from patients, perceptions of being at risk of malpractice complaints, clinical uncertainty, lack of a sense of competence, compulsion to "do something" and failure to keep up with advances in treatment such as sumatriptan for migraine.

A tailored implementation strategy to improve the management of headache by primary care physicians and reduce unnecessary referrals might include traineeships at headache clinics in a neurology department, including supervised, "hands-on" practice with patients' information to reduce misperceptions about liability risks and increase confidence in not referring patients, practical guidelines for investigating and counselling patients supported by local opinion leaders and appropriate patient information.

Low-risk patients with little or no potential for benefit may be screened for high blood cholesterol while high risk patients with a potential to benefit may not be screened due to patient expectations, failure of clinicians to remember to screen high-risk patients, reluctance of clinicians to not screen low-risk patients who request the test, local standards of practice, opinion leaders, medical training and advocacy.

An intervention to overcome these barriers might be to mail a simple set of six questions to patients that would characterise their risk of coronary heart disease, advising patients that those who score high (above whatever threshold is used) should be tested for high blood cholesterol and those who score low should not need to be tested.

Box 8.5 Evaluating implementation strategies

Types of evaluation	Examples
RCT randomised by patient	For implementation strategies where there is unlikely to be a learning or carry-over effect, such as mailing advice about cholesterol screening to patients, randomisation of patients may be appropriate. However, for most implementation strategies, randomisation by patient where individual clinicians see patients in both the experimental and control groups, RCTs randomised by patient are likely to be "contaminated" and result in underestimation of the effects of the strategy.
RCT randomised by provider	Randomisation by clinicians, for example in a trial of strategies to improve screening and counselling for alcohol misuse, may also be at risk of "contamination" if clinicians in the same practice are in both the experimental and control groups. This may be less of a problem if the effect is unlikely to carry over from one clinician to another; for example, for skills training for a procedure like proctoscopy. When clinicians rather than patients are randomised it is important that the analysis takes this into account to avoid unit of analysis errors.[35]
RCT randomised by groups of providers	Randomising by groups of providers, such as practices, hospitals, or communities, minimises the risk of contamination but also reduces the power of an evaluation and increases the risk of a confounder (such as a particularly influential clinician in one of the groups) biasing the results (despite randomisation) if there are too few units randomised. For example, in a "firm study" patients might be randomised to one ward (or practice) or another with only two "firms". This study would have, in effect, only two units of analysis. Although it was randomised, it may be difficult to disentangle the effects of the particular clinicians in the two firms from the effects of the intervention (for example, audio and feedback to reduce unnecessary use of laboratory or radiological tests).
Cross-over trial	As with RCTs where patients are randomised, for implementation strategies where there is unlikely to be a learning or carry-over effect, such as a comparison of computer-assisted drug dosage with non-computer-assisted drug dosage, a cross-over trial may be appropriate and increase the power of the study. However, for most implementation strategies there is likely to be an "order effect" in a cross-over trial if the intervention is effective which may make the results difficult to interpret.
Balanced block design	This study has the advantages of RCTs randomised by group (assuming group randomisation is used) and at the same time can reduce the potential of a "Hawthorne effect" (see p. 108). For example, clinicians within practices might be randomised to a traineeship for either headache or low back pain and be in the control group for the other clinical problem.
Before-after study	Before–after studies, for example, recording the provision of preventive services before and after an intervention such as using structured forms in patient records, are generally easy to conduct and common. However, they are highly susceptible to bias. Because they do not control for potential confounders, in particular changes occurring over time independently of the intervention (but also changes associated with the intervention, such as how data are recorded), they are often difficult or impossible to interpret. Indeed, the magnitude of bias is often as large or larger than the size of the expected changes in practice. In general, before–after studies are likely to overestimate effectiveness, but the size and even the direction of the bias cannot be known with certainty.
Interrupted time series analysis	Although interrupted time series analyses have some of the same limitations as before–after studies, they can under some circumstances provide reliable data if they are conducted on a large scale, for example to measure the effects of disseminating clinical practice guidelines on a national level when routinely collected data (for example, regarding Caesarean section rates)[19] are available that reliably reflect what is done in practice.

than doctors in the control group, with the result that the evaluation may overestimate the true effects of guidelines.

Cross-over trials,[15] in which clinicians act as their own controls receiving different interventions in random order, can be a powerful design. However, because there may be contamination across periods due to (for example) learning effects, the evaluation may underestimate the effect of implementation.

Balanced block design is attractive for evaluating implementation strategies in which each participating health care professional experiences both an implementation strategy (for one or more clinical problems) and the status quo (for one or more other clinical problems) simultaneously.[16] Such designs, in which health care professionals are randomised either individually or in groups, are likely to provide the most reliable evidence.[17]

Before–after studies with non-randomised controls that compare changes in the targeted behaviour with a control group of activities performed by study doctors but not targeted by guidelines[18] may provide useful though less reliable results. Before–after studies controlled by data from other sites are more robust if baseline characteristics and performance in control and study sites are similar, and data collection is contemporaneous in study and control sites during both phases of the study. Simple, uncontrolled before and after study designs where secular trends or sudden changes make it impossible to attribute observed changes to the intervention are not reliable.[17]

Interrupted time series analyses can be used to analyse before–after data in an attempt to detect whether an intervention has had an effect significantly greater than the underlying trend.[19] Such analyses can be useful, particularly when randomisation is not practical, provided that reliable data are available for objective measures of practice or health care outcomes, the intervention is independent of other changes, data collection is the same before and after the intervention, and formal tests of trend are used with a sufficient number of data points (at least 12) before and after the intervention.[9]

The need for collaboration

Over the past 20 years the development of explicit practice guidelines has increased dramatically. These efforts have been organised under a variety of rubrics, including quality assurance, total quality management, continuous quality improvement, technology assessment, outcomes management, audit and continuing medical education. To a large extent, all of these efforts have had similar goals. Provided guidelines are valid, whatever they are called, the growth in efforts to develop them could make an important contribution to improving the quality of care. However, there are potential problems. First, the methods for developing guidelines vary widely and the extent to which they are based on available scientific evidence is uncertain. Second, conflicting recommendations from different groups may lead to confusion, aggravation, general mistrust of guidelines, and even demoralisation and nihilism. Furthermore, although the independent development of consistent guidelines might be considered reassuring, it might also represent unnecessary duplication of effort and wasted resources. Third, the overall pattern of guideline development may not adequately reflect priorities for primary health care as a whole; there are likely important areas in which guideline development is lacking. Fourth, a profusion of guidelines may overwhelm clinicians and adversely affect the dissemination and use of guidelines. Most organisations producing guidelines have not adequately addressed implementation. Simply producing a guideline is unlikely to improve practice and benefit patients if active steps are not taken to ensured their appropriate use.[8,10,20]

Collaboration and coordination of efforts to develop and implement evidence-based clinical practice guidelines are essential.[21] It is unreasonable to expect health care professionals to manage scientific information and quality assurance independently.[21,22] It is beyond the capacity of individual physicians to independently access all the scientific information they need, measure their performance, and then design and evaluate strategies for improving their performance when it is sub-optimal. They lack the time, resources and often the necessary skills for these activities. Even if clinicians could independently undertake these activities, there would be a tremendous amount of unnecessary duplication of effort and inefficiency in such an approach. There is a clear need for organised programmes to assist physicians, other health care providers, consumers and others to manage scientific information and apply it in practice. Such programmes should include the following.

An advisory committee

Both the theory of diffusion of innovations and the social influences model of behaviour change suggest that opinion leaders transmit norms and model appropriate behaviour. Involving them in programmes to implement evidence-based care has the potential to promote change in health care provider performance.[23-25] A first step in organising a programme to implement evidence-based care might be to form an advisory committee composed, to some extent, of opinion leaders in primary care.

There is a great deal of variation in the potential to identify opinion leaders and in the potential of opinion leaders to influence practice among communities, within communities among clinicians and among clinical problems for the same clinician.[26] Nonetheless, through a survey and "snowballing" it may be possible to identify potential members of an advisory group within a region or on a national level who have the qualities desired of advisory group members and, at the same time, have qualities identified as important for opinion leaders.[26]

The advisory committee can assist in priority setting, guideline development and design of implementation strategies. If members of the advisory committee are opinion leaders, they can also form a component of some implementation strategies as "educational influentials".

Recruitment of participating providers

Consideration must be given to how to involve clinicians in a programme to implement evidence-based care. Clinical autonomy is highly valued by many clinicians, even if that autonomy translates into the right to provide care that conflicts with best evidence. Also, many clinicians are sceptical of organised efforts to improve their practice, often with good reason.[27] Establishment of an advisory group composed of peers who are respected by their colleagues (opinion leaders) can help to establish collaborative efforts. Other strategies that can be used include beginning with colleagues who are already enthusiastic, establishing explicit objectives that make clear the relevance and importance of the programme to clinicians, ensuring that the programme is "well oiled" and that participants do not lose precious time unnecessarily, establishing a non-threatening atmosphere, ensuring respect for individual clinicians and assuring confidentiality.

Establishment of priorities

The potential to provide health care will always be limited by the availability of resources. Consequently, choices must be made, either explicitly or implicitly, about priorities. This applies to decisions about programmes to improve the quality of care as well as to decisions about what care to provide to whom. Explicit criteria and processes to set priorities can help to protect against bias, arbitrary decisions and disagreement. Criteria that can be used to identify and select clinical problems to be targeted include the frequency of the problem, the severity of the problem, the availability of evidence to guide how the problem should be managed, the availability of indicators to measure practice and indications of variation in how the problem is currently managed.[27] Existing, readily available data together with input from the advisory committee can be used to set priorities. The priority-setting process can be designed to be expedient, relying heavily on the expertise of the members of the advisory committee (Box 8.6).

Guidelines development

The core element of systematically developed, evidence-based practice guidelines is a systematic review of the available comparative evidence. There is more likely to be agreement (consensus) if good research evidence

---

Box 8.6   Examples of priority-setting criteria*

Organisation	Criteria

US Institute of Medicine	Objective
	    Prevalence of the condition
	    Cost of technology
	    Variation in use of the technology
	Subjective
	    Burden of illness
	    Potential to change health outcomes
	    Potential to change costs
	    Potential to clarify ethical, legal, or social issues

College of Family Physicians of Canada	Frequency of condition Seriousness of health consequences Effect of intervention
American College of Physicians	Potential significant health benefit Potential risk Potential wide application Extent of interest to practitioners
American Medical Association	Potential impact on substantial patient population Controversy within the medical community Availability of scientific data

* Criteria for technology assessment or development of clinical practice guidelines[27]

---

is available,[28–30] and it can be argued that it is dangerous to attempt to reach a consensus that goes beyond the available evidence.[31]

Because undertaking a systematic review may be the most demanding aspect of preparing valid practice guidelines, consideration should be given to using existing reviews, particularly Cochrane Reviews.[32] If a Cochrane Review is not available, consideration should be given to preparing a review as a Cochrane Review. Using or preparing a Cochrane Review can help to avoid unnecessary duplication of effort, ensure the comprehensiveness of the search for best current evidence, ensure the validity of the review in other ways[33] and provide a mechanism for keeping the review up to date.

As noted in the beginning of this chapter, a systematic review of the evidence is essential but not sufficient to make a rational decision about how to manage a health care problem. Other types of information and judgements are also necessary. An advisory committee can help to ensure that other types of information (about needs, resources and preferences) are taken into account and that the judgements that are made in reaching a conclusion are sensible in the context of the primary care setting in which the recommendations that are made will be implemented.

Assessment of current practice

Once it is determined what should be done based on current best evidence, it is necessary to determine whether current practice is evidence-based.[34] Existing sources of data, particularly computerised journals and centralised databases (for example, for laboratory test ordering, prescribing, or referrals) should be used as far as possible. Additional low-cost methods of collecting data on performance may be developed and employed; for example, use of duplicate prescriptions or test ordering forms, or simple registers maintained by laboratories, pharmacies, or hospitals.

Development of implementation strategies

When sub-optimal practice is identified and quality improvement efforts are warranted, specific quality improvement strategies should be designed based on an assessment of the underlying causes of the sub-optimal care, as discussed above.

Evaluation of implementation strategies

Dramatic changes in practice are likely to be rare. Most often, changes will be moderate at best[8] and rigorous evaluation is needed to determine whether efforts to improve care are effective. Ideally, participating practices should be randomly allocated to receive each implementation strategy or act as a control. For evaluations of each strategy, the unit of analysis should be the participating practice. The main outcome measures should be objectively measured performance in the participating practices. Sample sizes should be calculated taking into account clustering.[35]

Evaluation of the programme

Uncoordinated, non-collaborative models of primary care (the current norm in most parts of the world) result in important gaps between evidence and practice, inefficient use of resources and harm. The need for programmes to implement evidence-based care seems obvious and the key elements of such programmes rest, to a large extent, on simple logic. However, the effectiveness and efficiency of such programmes cannot be assumed. Ongoing, rigorous evaluations of the effectiveness of the implementation strategies that are used will provide a solid basis for evaluating the overall effectiveness of such programmes. In addition, evaluation of programmes to implement evidence-based care should include an economic analysis of their overall cost-effectiveness, and provider and consumer satisfaction should be measured as well as effectiveness in changing professional practice and improving health care outcomes.

Getting started

In the absence of an organised programme to implement evidence-based care, what can individual clinicians do to improve the use of evidence in their practices? The starting point for implementing evidence must be critical reflection: awareness of discomfort in a consultation and a sense of uncertainty. Unfortunately, many clinicians appear to lack this or alleviate their discomfort with uncertainty by avoiding critical reflection. For those clinicians who have acknowledged the need to improve the use of evidence in their practices, a good starting point may be to establish a small group of colleagues to provide a forum for support, critical reflection and carrying out the practical steps of implementing the evidence: setting priorities, determining how clinical problems should be managed, measuring and improving performance.[27] The next step is to acquire and apply critical appraisal skills. A growing set of resources is available to assist with this, including Internet sites, electronic databases and evidence-based journals that make high quality evidence more accessible, and users' guides published in journals and textbooks (see Chapter 3). To ensure that the evidence is implemented, it is necessary to develop simple mechanisms of monitoring what is done in practice. For this to be done efficiently, computerised medical records are important, if not essential. Clinicians who have computerised medical records should demand that the vendors of the software they use should provide tools to enable easily implemented audits, if they do not already have these.[37] When gaps are identified between what is being done and what should be done based on the evidence, discussing this with a small group of colleagues can help to identify the reasons for the gaps, barriers to reduce the gaps and strategies to overcome the barriers and implement the evidence. Visiting each other's practices can further help to identify barriers and design well tailored implementation strategies. Finally, to close the loop and ensure that the desired changes were, in fact, achieved, what is being done in practice needs to be monitored after implementing the evidence (Box 8.7).

Acknowledgements

Preparation of this chapter was supported in part by the Norwegian Medical Association Quality Assurance Fund.

Box 8.7   Getting started

Although organised programmes to implement evidence based care are needed, it is possible for small groups of clinicians to implement change on their own. For example, in two large academic group practices we were able to generate 30–40 evidence based practice guidelines per year, conduct 15–20 audits, and develop implementation strategies for a number of clinical problems where we found inconsistencies between the results of audits and evidence based guidelines.

Most of this work was undertaken by residents (physicians in specialty training in family medicine) under the supervision of one of the authors. Meetings were held once weekly for one hour, organised on a two or three monthly cycle. At the first meeting of each cycle we would identify clinical problems where clinical practice guidelines were needed and set priorities. The residents would then work in pairs to identify relevant evidence (preferably existing, systematically developed, clinical practice guidelines or systematic reviews) and critically appraise it, as a rule not using more than two hours for this. The best evidence that could be found would be copied circulated to everyone in the group and discussed. The pairs of residents would then draft guidelines based on the evidence and discussion using a structured format,[7] which would subsequently be presented and discussed by the clinical faculty.

Although this approach did not always result in adequate guidelines due to the limited amount of time and resources available, it frequently led to the identification of clear recommendations supported by good evidence. Frequently, when the residents conducted chart audits to find out what was being done in practice, we found discrepancies between what we concluded we should be doing and what we were doing in practice.[34,36]

Using this approach, residents were able to find and critically appraise evidence competently for problems raised in the group, and we often were able to identify likely barriers to improving practice and generate possible strategies for overcoming those barriers. However, residents and others in the practices did not find time to apply these skills outside of this structured approach and we generally were not able to implement or evaluate the strategies that we developed. The latter is difficult at best within an individual practice and requires the collaboration of multiple practices, as discussed in the text.

References

1 Egger M, Smith GD, Altman DG. eds. *Systematic reviews in health care. Meta-analysis in context*. London: BMJ Publishing Group, 2001.

2 Glasziou P, Irwig L. An evidence-based approach to individualising patient treatment. *BMJ* 1995;**311**:1356–9.

3 Smith R. What clinical information do doctors need? *BMJ* 1996;1062–8.

4 Armstrong D, Fry J, Armstrong P. Doctors' perceptions of pressure from patients for referral. *BMJ* 1991;**302**:1186–8.

5 Woodward CA, Rosser W. Effect of medico-legal liability on patterns of general and family practice in Canada. *Can Med Assoc J* 1989;**141**:291–9.

6 Eddy DM. Clinical policies and the quality of clinical practice. *N Engl J Med* 1982;**307**:343–7.

7 Oxman AD, Feightner JW, for the Evidence Based Care Resource Group. Evidence-based care. 2. Setting guidelines: how should we manage this problem? *Can Med Assoc J* 1994;**150**:1417-23.

8 Oxman AD, Thomson AD, Davis DA, Haynes RB. No magic bullets: a systematic review of 102 trials of interventions to improve professional practice. *Can Med Assoc J* 1995;**153**:1423-31.

9 Bero L, Grilli R, Grimshaw J, Oxman A, Zwarebstein M, eds. Cochrane effective practice and organisation of care module. In: *Cochrane Collaboration. Cochrane Library*. Oxford: Update Software, 2000, 4.

10 Bero L, Grilli R, Grimshaw J, Harvey E, Oxman AD, Thomson MA. Getting research findings into practice: closing the gap between research and practice: an overview of systematic reviews of interventions to promote the implementation of research findings. *BMJ* 1998;**317**:465-8.

11 Getting evidence into practice. *Effective Health Care* 1999;**5**(1):1-16.

12 Avorn J, Sournerai SB. Improving drug-therapy decisions through educational research outreach. A randomised controlled trial of academically based "detailing". *N Engl J Med* 1983;**24**:1457-63.

13 Morgan M, Studney DR, Barnett GO, *et al*. Computerised concurrent review of prenatal care. *Qual Rev Bull* 1978;**4**:33-6.

14 Moser CA, Kalton G. *Survey methods in social investigation*, 2nd edn. Aldershot: Gower, 1971.

15 Landgren FT, Harvey KJ, Mashford ML, *et al*. Changing antibiotic prescribing by educational marketing. *Med J Aust* 1988;**149**:595-9.

16 Norton PG, Dempsey LJ. Self-audit: its effect on quality of care. *J Fam Pract* 1985;**21**:289-91.

17 Effective Health Care. *Implementing clinical guidelines. Can guidelines be used to improve clinical practice?* Bulletin No 8. Leeds: University of Leeds, 1994.

18 De Vos Meiring P, Wells IR. The effect of radiology guidelines for general practitioners in Plymouth. *Clin Radiol* 1990;**42**:327-9.

19 Lornas J, Anderson GM, Domnick-Pierre K, Vayda E, Enkin MW, Hannah WJ. Do practice guidelines guide practice? The effect of a consensus statement on the practice of physicians. *N Engl J Med* 1989;**321**:1306-11.

20 Grimshaw JM, Russell IT. Effect of clinical guidelines on medical practice: a systematic review of rigorous evaluations. *Lancet* 1993;**342**:1317-22.

21 Oxman AD. Coordination of guidelines development. *Can Med Assoc J* 1993;**148**:1285-8.

22 Williamson M, German PS, Weiss R, Skinner EA, Bowes F. Health science information management and continuing education of physicians. *Ann Intern Med* 1989;**110**:151-60.

23 Greer AL. The state of the art versus the state of the science: the diffusion of new medical technologies into practice. *Int J Tech Assess Health Care* 1988;**4**:5-26.

24 Mittman BS, Tonesk X, Jacobson PD. Implementing clinical practice guidelines: social influence strategies and practitioner behaviour change. *Qual Rev Bull* 1992; **18**:413-22.

25 Lomas J, Enkin MW, Anderson GM, Harmah WJ, Vayda E, Singer J. Opinion leaders vs audit and feedback to implement practice guidelines: delivery after previous caesarean section. *JAMA* 1991;**265**:2202-7.

26 Flottorp S, Oxman AD, Bjørndal A. The limits of leadership: opinion leaders in general practice. *J Health Serv Res Policy* 1998;**3**:197-202.

27 Oxman AD, MacDonald PJ, for the Evidence-Based Care Resource Group. Evidence based care. 1. Setting priorities: how important is this problem? *Can Med Assoc J* 1994;**150**:1249-54.

28 Brook RH, Park RE, Winslow CM, *et al.* Diagnosis and treatment of coronary disease: comparison of doctors' attitudes in the USA and the UK. *Lancet* 1988;1(8588):750–3.

29 Jacoby I. Evidence and consensus. *JAMA* 1988;**259**:3039.

30 Lomas J, Anderson G, Enkin M, Vayda E, Roberts R, MacKinnon B. The role of evidence in the consensus process: results from a Canadian consensus exercise. *JAMA* 1988;**259**:3001–5.

31 Williams C. The value of consensus. *Eur J Cancer* 1991;27:525–6.

32 Cochrane database of systematic reviews. In: *Cochrane Collaboration. Cochrane Library*. Oxford: Update Software, 2000, 4.

33 Clarke M, Oxman AD, eds. Improving and updating reviews. In: *The Cochrane reviewers' handbook*, section 10. *Cochrane Library*. Oxford: Update Software, 2000, 4.

34 Hutchison BG, Feightner JW, Lusk S, for the Evidence Based Care Resource Group. Evidence-based care. 3. Measuring performance: how are we managing this problem? *Can Med Assoc J* 1994;**150**:1575–9.

35 Whiting-O'Keefe QE, Henke C, Simborg DW. Choosing the correct unit of analysis in medical care experiments. *Med Care* 1984;**22**:1101–14.

36 Oxman AD, Davis DA, for the Evidence Based Care Resource Group. Evidence-based care. 4. Improving performance: how can we improve the way we manage this problem? *Can Med Assoc J* 1994;**150**:1793–6.

37 Treweek S, Flottorp S, Oxman A. Improving the quality of primary care through tailored interventions and customisable software linked to electronic medical records. *Health Informatics J* 2000;**6**:212–18.

9: Identifying and using evidence-based guidelines in general practice

JEREMY GRIMSHAW AND MARTIN ECCLES

Introduction

Clinical guidelines are "systematically developed statements to assist practitioner and patient decisions about appropriate health care for specific clinical circumstances".[1] They are increasingly seen as a source of clinical information to answer questions formulated by individual professionals: Guyatt and Rennie,[2] in the editorial accompanying the Users' Guide to Medical Literature series in the *Journal of the American Medical Association* (JAMA), suggested that "resolving a clinical problem begins with a search for a *valid* overview (systematic review) or practice guideline as the most efficient method of deciding on the best patient care". Guidelines are considered valid if "when followed they lead to the health gains and costs predicted for them".[1] Guidelines are more likely to be valid if they are based on systematic literature reviews, are produced by national or regional guideline development groups that include representatives of all key disciplines, and if the links between recommendations and scientific evidence are made explicit.[3,4] Unfortunately, there are many guidelines available of variable quality and it is therefore important that practitioners are able to appraise a guideline before deciding whether to follow its recommendations.[5]

We envisage three possible scenarios in which general practitioners could use clinical guidelines to support their practice. Firstly, general practitioners may use guidelines as an information source for continuing professional educational activities. Valid clinical guidelines provide an up-to-date broad overview of the management of a condition or the use of an intervention; as such they provide an important source of information for continuing professional education activities. In this context, we would argue that guidelines have potential advantages over systematic reviews. Guidelines usually have a broader scope than systematic reviews, which tend to focus on an individual problem or intervention. They may also provide a more coherent integrated view on how to manage a condition. The broader issues within continuing professional education are discussed in Chapter 11.

Secondly, general practitioners may use guidelines to answer specific clinical questions arising out of their day-to-day practice. A key step is to frame the clinical question of interest in such a way that it can be answered, specifying the patient or problem, the intervention of interest and possible comparison interventions and the outcomes of interest (see Sackett *et al.*[6] for a further discussion of this). This allows the general practitioner to identify what sort of evidence to search for. Under these circumstances, we would argue that clinical guidelines are only one of many types of evidence that are potentially relevant (for example, if the general practitioner is interested in a question relating to the effectiveness of an intervention, he or she should also search for relevant systematic reviews). These issues are discussed in further detail in Chapters 2–6.

Thirdly, general practitioners, practices or area-wide organisations (for example, primary care groups and trusts) may use guidelines as tools within quality improvement activities within a single general practice or across a number of practices.[7] In this context, the broad integrated scope of guidelines have advantages over other evidence sources.

The first section of this chapter considers how to identify clinical guidelines, then how to appraise them (important first steps common to all three scenarios) and finally discusses the issues that general practitioners should consider if they wish to implement guidelines within quality improvement activities in their practices.

Identifying practice guidelines

Identifying clinical guidelines is problematical for two reasons. Firstly, many guidelines are published in the grey literature and are not indexed in the commonly available bibliographic databases (although there are a number of bibliographic databases available which specialise in grey literature). For example none of the guidelines published by the Agency for Health Care Policy and Research are identifiable on MEDLINE. Secondly, even if guidelines are published in indexed journals, optimal search strategies have not yet been developed: in the Ovid version of MEDLINE,[8] practice guidelines can be identified under a variety of headings including: *guideline* (publication type), *practice guideline* (publication type), *practice guidelines* (MeSH heading), *Consensus Development Conference* (publication type) and *Consensus Development Conference, NIH* (publication type). A preliminary examination in several clinical areas suggests that *guideline* (publication type) is probably the most sensitive and specific individual search term (See Appendix 1 for a sample MEDLINE search strategy that can be used when looking for guidelines.)

Fortunately, there are a number of other resources available to help practitioners, in particular there are a number of sites on the Internet that catalogue clinical guidelines. Full text versions or abstracts of guidelines are available from some sites (see Box 9.1 for some currently available sites we find useful). It is likely that such sites will become the best source to identify guidelines in the future. Another strategy which general practitioners could consider is to develop a practice library of valid clinical guidelines by appraising any guidelines they are sent.

Box 9.1   Electronic guideline resources

Australian National Health and Medical Research Council (NHMRC) – full text versions of guidelines and other resources (www.health.gov.au/nhmrc/publicat/cp-home.htm)

Canadian Medical Association Clinical Practice Guidelines Infobase – index of clinical practice guidelines, including downloadable full text versions or abstracts of most guidelines (www.cma.ca/cpgs/index.html)

National Institute for Clinical Excellence – full text versions of guidelines and other resources (www.nice.org.uk)

New Zealand Guidelines Group – full text versions of guidelines and other resources (www.nzgg.org.nz/library.htm)

Scottish Intercollegiate Guidelines Network – full text versions of guidelines and other resources (www.show.scot.nhs.uk/sign/graphic.htm)

US National Guidelines Clearing House – index of clinical guidelines including structured synopsis of development methods and key recommendations (www.guideline.gov/index.asp)

(Note: at the time of writing the electronic addresses given are correct, however these are liable to change over time.)

Appraising practice guidelines

There are many potential biases inherent in guideline development which need to be overcome to ensure the validity of the resulting guideline. When a general practitioner has identified a relevant guideline, it is important that he or she appraises its validity before deciding whether to adopt its recommendations.[5] If general practitioners adopt invalid guideline recommendations, this may lead to wasteful use of resources on ineffective interventions or, even worse, harm to patients.

A number of checklists for guideline appraisal have been proposed. Field and Lohr[9] proposed a draft appraisal instrument for clinical guidelines, however, Cluzeau and colleagues[10] found this difficult to use in practice and developed a shorter version which is currently being evaluated.[11] Both of these instruments are probably more relevant to national or regional appraisal of guidelines, but may be useful for general practitioners and practices when identifying guidelines for quality improvement activities.

General practitioners seeking to identify valid guidelines for their own purposes may prefer a briefer and more practical approach to appraisal. We would suggest that general practitioners should not consider guidelines which fail to report development methods explicitly by including a methods section within the guideline or supporting papers (see Eccles *et al.*[12] for an example). Although using this as a filter would exclude many guidelines currently developed and disseminated in the UK, we would argue that without such information it is impossible to appraise the validity of guidelines and, as a result, it is difficult to have confidence in a guideline's recommendations.

The Users' Guides to the Medical Literature series included three papers on appraising and using clinical guidelines[13-15]: they propose a series of primary and secondary guides or questions to help practitioners appraise a guideline (Box 9.2). The primary questions act as a filter to determine whether practitioners should consider the guideline recommendations. General practitioners should use their clinical judgement to assess whether all reasonable practice options and important outcomes have been considered. They should then consider the guideline development methods used with particular *emphasis* on the methods chosen to identify, select and combine evidence. Guidelines are more likely to be valid if the developers have used a systematic review to identify relevant evidence. If guideline developers fail to report their search methods explicitly it is difficult to assess whether they are likely to have identified all of the relevant evidence. If guideline developers have reported their search methods, general practitioners need to consider whether the search terms were comprehensive or whether there were important gaps that may lead to invalid recommendations. If general practitioners cannot convince themselves that a comprehensive systematic review has been undertaken during guideline development, they should not consider a guideline further.

Box 9.2   Guides for appraising guidelines. From Hayward *et al.*[13]

Primary guides
Were all important options and outcomes clearly stated?
Was an explicit and sensible process used to identify, select and combine evidence?

Secondary guides
Was an explicit and sensible process used to consider the relative value of different outcomes?
Is the guideline likely to account for important recent developments?
Has the guideline been subject to peer review and testing?

In addition to the questions identified by the Users' Guides to the Medical Literature papers, we would add two further questions that general practitioners should consider when appraising guidelines. Firstly, was the guideline development group multidisciplinary with adequate representation from primary care? Guideline recommendations are influenced by the knowledge and values of the development group members.[16] Therefore it is reasonable to expect that guidelines intended for use in primary care should have an appropriate representation of primary health care professionals within the group. Secondly, do the guidelines present explicit links between recommendations and the evidence supporting them? In most guidelines, the strength of evidence supporting individual recommendations will vary; some recommendations will be supported by a substantial and consistent body of evidence derived from rigorous studies, whereas other recommendations will be supported by expert opinion alone. It is important that the end users of a guideline are aware of the strength of supporting evidence as this may influence whether they choose to follow an individual recommendation or not (for example, an end user should have good grounds for not following a recommendation based upon rigorously derived evidence). The use of explicit links between evidence and recommendation makes the process of deriving a recommendation more explicit for the end user. There are a number of systems of increasing sophistication available for expressing the strength of evidence and grade of recommendation (see Box 9.3 for an example). We would suggest that guidelines which use such a system are more likely to be valid and are more likely to be useful to general practitioners.

Implementing clinical practice guidelines within the process of quality improvement in general practice

The introduction identified three scenarios in which general practitioners could use clinical guidelines to support their practice: as educational materials for continuing professional development activities; as a type of evidence to answer specific clinical questions; and as a focus for quality improvement activities in the practice. The process of identifying and appraising guidelines was common to all three scenarios. This section considers the processes involved in implementing clinical practice guidelines within the process of quality improvement in general practice. This is conceptualised as a series of steps that move from the identification of a relevant guideline through the process of local adaptation to the implementation and monitoring of the practice guideline. Whilst these steps have been described in generic terms they require implementation within specific health care systems. Thus in the UK the appropriate "unit" for such activities may, for some topics, still be the individual general

Box 9.3 Levels of evidence and grades of guideline recommendations

Levels of evidence

Level	Type of evidence – description[17]
Ia	Evidence obtained from meta-analysis of randomised trials
Ib	Evidence obtained from at least one randomised trial
IIa	Evidence obtained from at least one well-designed controlled study without randomisation
IIb	Evidence obtained from at least one other type of well-designed quasi-experimental study
III	Evidence obtained from well-designed, non-experimental descriptive studies, such as comparative studies, correlation studies and case studies
IV	Evidence obtained from expert committee reports or opinions or clinical experiences of respected authorities

Grades of guideline recommendations

Grade	Nature of recommendation
A	Based on clinical studies of good quality and consistency addressing the specific recommendation and including at least one randomised trial
B	Based on well-conducted clinical studies but without randomised clinical trials on the topic of the recommendation
C	Made despite the absence of directly applicable clinical studies of good quality

practice. However, in a climate of policy changes where clinical topics are the subject of initiatives such as the UK NHS "National Service Frameworks", it is increasingly likely that quality improvement activities will be conducted in common across general practices as well as within them. Structures such as primary care groups and primary care trusts facilitate such developments. While this may increase the scale and complexity of some of the tasks the underlying principles remain true.

Practice based quality improvement system

For the majority of clinical conditions in general practice, the administration and provision of health care is dependent upon a multidisciplinary practice team. As a result, it is important to plan guideline implementation and quality improvement activities from a multidisciplinary perspective. We would suggest that practices wishing to implement guidelines within a process of quality improvement should develop a co-ordinating mechanism for these activities. It is likely that this would involve the establishment of a co-ordinating group, which should be appropriately multidisciplinary to allow the views of all relevant stakeholders to be represented and also to draw on the full range of skills available within a practice. For example, such a group could include administrative, medical and nursing input. Depending on the particular topic this group may be solely within one practice or working across a group of practices.

The group could be responsible for prioritisation of topics and negotiations about allocation of resources to support quality improvement activities. A single general practice will only be able to deal with a limited number of guideline implementation activities at any one point in time. Therefore practices should prioritise topics for quality improvement based upon perceived problems in the practice. In general, practices should concentrate upon clinical areas: with high morbidity, disability or mortality; where effective treatments are available; where there is a perception that the practice is not achieving optimal levels of care; and where there are existing rigorously developed guidelines available for adaptation. Practices may also need to give priority to clinical areas where there is an existing area-wide quality improvement programme (for example, co-ordinated by primary care group structures) with supporting materials already developed.

Quality improvement activities involving guideline implementation have financial and human costs. For example, most implementation activities will involve resources associated with staff time to allow their participation in adaptation and implementation of guidelines, the specific costs of the implementation strategies, and staff costs associated with monitoring implementation. In some cases, implementation of guidelines may have considerable resource implications. For example, when considering the implementation of hypertension guidelines, a practice may decide to establish a nurse-run clinic for routine monitoring of patients. This would require the practice to either find new resources to increase nursing time or reallocate existing resources. The co-ordinating group would need to identify potential resource implications of implementing guidelines and negotiate for resources within the practice.

Adapting valid guidelines

Few practices have the resources or skills to develop their own valid evidence-based guidelines. Therefore we would recommend that practices should identify an existing rigorously developed guideline rather than attempt to develop de novo guidelines.[7] The process of identifying and appraising guidelines has already been discussed. In this section, the process of guideline adaptation within a practice is considered. In general, this should follow the same principles used to increase the likelihood of valid guideline development.[4] The adaptation group should include all relevant stakeholders from within (and without) the practice; the membership should also encompass the range of individuals who will be needed to complete the implementation and evaluation of the guideline. In addition, the group undertaking the process needs to ensure that, between them, they can fulfil the necessary roles that may be required: specialist resource; group leadership; administrative support. Whilst members of the practice may be able to fulfil some of these roles, external advisers may need to be brought in. For example, if a practice is adapting a guideline for the management of dementia they may seek specialist input from a psychiatrist with special interest in psychiatric disorders of the elderly (psycho-geriatrician).

Two main factors will influence how a guideline is adapted by a local group: the strength of recommendation within the guideline and local circumstances. As a result of the subjective element involved in the interpretation of evidence when deriving recommendations, there is always the potential for a group to re-interpret evidence and derive different recommendations. Deciding whether or not to derive different recommendations should be based, in large part, on the nature of the supporting evidence. Local adaptation groups should be wary of changing recommendations based upon good evidence but have greater freedom to change recommendations based upon weak evidence. Where recommendations based on good evidence are changed the reasons for this should be explicitly acknowledged.

Local circumstances may influence whether a recommendation is practicable or how it can be achieved. For example, the North of England Evidence Based Guideline on Stable Angina[18] recommends that all patients should have an exercise tolerance test, a recommendation based upon good evidence. However, this may not be achievable if practices are located in an area where their local hospital does not have exercise testing facilities.

Implementing practice based guidelines

There are a number of barriers to the implementation of practice based guidelines which may operate at a system or individual level (see Lomas[19] for further discussion of barriers to implementation; see also Chapters 8 and 12). As a result, the production of a practice based guideline is usually insufficient by itself to ensure implementation of guideline recommendations.

The co-ordination group should attempt to identify potential barriers to implementation during the practice based guideline development process. Potential barriers may exist if, for example: the practice does not have access to an external resource (for example, if a practice does not have easy access to exercise testing when attempting to implement practice based guidelines for angina); the practice does not have the necessary internal systems (for example, a disease register when attempting to implement practice based guidelines to prevent loss to follow up of hypertensive patients); the health care professionals involved in the management of the condition are unaware of the desired changes (for example, if the health care professionals have not managed to keep up to date with recent research findings); if health care professionals fail to recognise that their performance is suboptimal; if the established culture, routines and practice of health care professionals opposes the desired changes; or if the health care professionals have problems processing and managing information in the consultation resulting in the omission of important activities (see McDonald[20] for further discussion). Frequently more than one barrier operating at different levels may be present.

The co-ordination group has to decide which barriers are the most important and decide upon strategies to overcome these. This may involve: negotiation with external bodies (for example, a practice may wish to discuss the establishment of an open access exercise testing service when implementing guidelines for angina); reorganisation of internal systems (for example, establishing a disease register for hypertensive patients); and targeting professional behaviour change strategies to address barriers at the level of the individual health care professional within the practice. There are a number of potential implementation strategies that may be used to ensure that health care professionals in a practice implement a guideline[21] (Box 9.4; also see Box 8.3). An overview of systematic reviews of professional behaviour change strategies noted that most reviews identified small to modest improvements in processes of care; the authors concluded that specific strategies to implement research-based recommendations appear necessary to ensure practice change, with existing studies suggesting that more intensive efforts to alter practice are generally more successful.[22]

In general, the choice of strategy should reflect the perceived barriers, the available resources for implementation and the ease of introducing the implementation strategy within the practice. Educational approaches (attendance at seminars and workshops) may be useful where barriers relate to health care professionals' knowledge. Audit and feedback may be useful when health care professionals are unaware of suboptimal practice. Social influence approaches (local consensus processes, educational outreach, opinion leaders, marketing, etc.) may be useful when barriers relate to the existing culture, routines and practices of health care professionals (see Mittman et al.[23] for further discussion). Reminders and patient-mediated interventions may be useful when health care professionals have problems processing information within consultations. Given that there are frequently several barriers to implementation, it is not surprising that multifaceted interventions are usually more effective than single interventions[24,25] (see Chapter 8 for further discussion of the need for tailoring of implementation strategies to address identified barriers).

Box 9.4 Interventions to promote professional behavioural change that could be used to implement research findings. From Bero *et al.*[21]

Educational materials – Distribution of published or printed recommendations for clinical care, including clinical practice guidelines, audio-visual materials and electronic publications. The materials may have been delivered personally or through personal or mass mailings.

Conferences – Participation of health care providers in conferences, lectures, workshops or traineeships.

Local consensus process – Inclusion of participating providers in discussion to ensure that they agree that the chosen clinical problem is important and the approach to managing the problem (i.e. the clinical practice guideline or definition of adequate care) is appropriate. The consensus process might also address the design of an intervention to improve performance.

Educational outreach visits – Use of a trained person who meets with providers in their practice settings to provide information with the intent of changing the providers' performance. The information given may include feedback on the providers' performance.

Local opinion leaders – Use of providers nominated by their colleagues as "educationally influential". The investigators must explicitly state that the opinion leaders were identified by their colleagues.

Patient mediated interventions – Any intervention aimed at changing the performance of health care providers where specific information was sought from or given to patients, for example, direct mailings to patients, patient counselling delivered by someone other than the targeted providers, clinical information collected from patients by others and given to the provider, educational materials given to patients or placed in waiting rooms.

Audit and feedback – Any summary of clinical performance over a specified period of time. Summarised information may include the average number of diagnostic tests ordered, the average cost per test or per patient, the average number of prescriptions written, the proportion of times a desired clinical action was taken, etc. The summary may also include recommendations for clinical care. The information may be given in a written or verbal format.

Reminders (manual or computerised) – Any intervention that prompts the health care provider to perform a patient specific clinical action.

Marketing – Use of personal interviewing, group discussion ("focus groups") or a survey of targeted providers to identify barriers to change and the subsequent design of an intervention that addresses these barriers.

Multifaceted interventions – Any intervention that includes two or more of the above.

Evaluating implementation

Having developed and implemented a practice based guideline, the practice may wish to evaluate whether this process has lead to improvements in the quality of care. Chapter 7 comprises a detailed discussion of methods used in the evaluation of the application of evidence. The essential components include the development of *review criteria* (defined as "systematically developed statements that can be used to assess specific health care decisions, services and outcomes"[26]), *performance measurements* (defined as "methods or instruments to estimate or monitor the extent to which the actions of a health care practitioner or provider conform to the clinical practice guideline"[26]) and *standards of care*. Figure 9.1 shows how these different elements are related: guidelines (which prospectively guide care) are the source of review criteria (which retrospectively assess care); performance measurement is the mechanism by which the evaluation of care is conducted; and standards of performance are the relevant levels of achievement. This should all be conducted within the cyclical process of quality improvement within the practice.

Box 9.5 summarises the desired characteristics of review criteria. An example of how such criteria could be derived and used, based on a recommendation from the North of England Evidence Based Stable Angina Guideline,[18] is shown in Box 9.6. However, not all guideline recommendations within a guideline will make good medical review criteria; Hadorn and colleagues[27] were only able to derive eight review criteria from a guideline containing 34 recommendations.

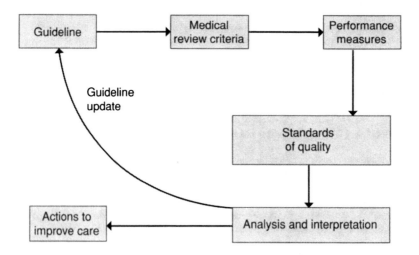

Fig 9.1 Deriving review criteria from guidelines. Adapted from Agency for Health Care Policy and Research.[26]

Box 9.5 Desirable characteristics of review criteria. Adapted from Agency for Health Care Policy and Research[26]

- **Sensitive** – if criterion classifies as conforming a high proportion that do conform

- **Specific** – if criterion classifies as non-conforming a high proportion that do not conform

- **Patient responsive** – allows some consideration of patient preference

- **Readable** – presented in language and format that can be understood by non-clinician reviewers

- **Minimally obtrusive** – criteria and process for applying them minimise inappropriate direct interaction with, and burdens on, the treating practitioner and patient

- **Feasible** – information for review can be obtained easily from providers, patients, records

- **Computer compatible** – readily transformed into computer protocols

- **Appeals criteria** – take explicit account of dealing with appeals against adverse decisions

---

Conclusions

This chapter has suggested a framework within which individual practices can identify, appraise and use guidelines to improve the quality of patient care. While guidelines can be used within continuing professional education and to answer questions identified during routine patient contacts, we have concentrated on how a practice could use a guideline within a system of quality improvement. In general, an individual general practice will not have the skills and resources available to develop *de novo* an evidence-based guideline. Instead, we suggest that practices should identify and adapt a valid guideline following a priority setting exercise. An integral part of this process is the identification of potential external, practice based and individually based barriers to implementation and multifaceted strategies to overcome these. Following this, a practice can derive review criteria to evaluate the effectiveness of their activities. Increasingly in the UK, area-wide primary care structures such as primary care groups or trusts will have a central role in supporting guideline implementation in practices.

Acknowledgements

The Health Services Research Unit is funded by the Chief Scientist Office of the Scottish Office Department of Health. However, the views expressed are those of the authors and not the funding body.

> **Box 9.6** Deriving review criteria, performance measures and standards from an evidence based guideline. Based upon North of England Stable Angina Guideline Development Group[18]
>
> **Relevant section of the guideline**
> SECONDARY PROPHYLACTIC TREATMENT
> Recommendation: All patients should be treated with aspirin in a daily dose of 75 mg (A[1]).
>
> *Statement: the use of aspirin in high-risk groups lowers the risk of subsequent vascular events (I[2]).*
>
> The AntiPlatelet Trialists' collaboration meta-analysis in 1994[28] demonstrated benefits for patients with angina being treated with aspirin. They analysed data on approximately 20 000 patients with suspected or definite acute myocardial infarction from nine trials (17 200 in ISIS 2). The rates of myocardial infarction (MI), stroke and vascular death in the anti-platelet group were 992/9388 (10.6%) compared with 1348/9385 (14.4%) in the controls, a 29% odds reduction (4% SD). This produced a reduction of 38/1000 in the risk of a subsequent vascular event. There was a similar picture from the other three high-risk groups: prior MI; prior stroke/transient ischaemic attack; other high-risk groups (unstable angina, stable angina, post coronary artery bypass graft).
>
> **Recommendation**
> All patients should be treated with aspirin in a daily dose of 75 mg
>
> **Review criteria**
> The patient was treated with aspirin in a daily dose of 75 mg
>
> **Performance measure**
> Number of cases treated/number of cases eligible
>
> **Standard**
> Performance rate of 80% or less triggers a review of the prescribing of secondary prophylactic treatment
>
> [1] Box 9.3 Grades of Guideline recommendations
> [2] Box 9.3 Levels of evidence

References

1 Institute of Medicine. In: Field MJ, Lohr KN, eds. *Guidelines for clinical practice. From development to use.* Washington: National Academy Press, 1992.

2 Guyatt G, Rennie D. Users' guides to the medical literature. *JAMA* 1993;270:2096–7.

3 Grimshaw JM, Russell IT. Achieving health gain through clinical guidelines. I: Developing scientifically valid guidelines. *Qual Health Care* 1993;2:243–8.

4 Grimshaw JM, Eccles MP, Russell IT. Developing clinically valid guidelines. *J Eval Clin Pract* 1995;1:37–48.

5 Cluzeau F, Littlejohns P, Grimshaw JM. Appraising clinical guidelines – towards a "Which?" guide for purchasers. *Qual Health Care* 1994;3:121–2.
6 Sackett DL, Richardson WS, Rosenberg W, Haynes RB. *Evidence-based medicine. How to practice and teach EBM.* New York: Churchill Livingstone, 1996.
7 Royal College of General Practitioners. *The development and implementation of clinical guidelines: report of the Clinical Guidelines Working Group.* Report from General Practice 26. London: Royal College of General Practitioners, 1996.
8 Ovid Technologies. *Ovid for Windows Version 3.0.* Ovid Technologies, 1996.
9 Field MJ, Lohr KN. Appendix B. A provisional instrument for assessing clinical practice guidelines. In Institute of Medicine, ed. *Guidelines for clinical practice. From development to use.* Washington: National Academy Press, 1992.
10 Cluzeau F, Littlejohns P, Grimshaw JM, Hopkins A. Appraising clinical guidelines and development of criteria: a pilot study. *J Interprofessional Care* 1995;9:227–35.
11 Cluzeau F, Littlejohns P, Grimshaw JM, Feder G, for Royal College of General Practitioners. Draft appraisal instrument for clinical guidelines (Appendix 1). In: *The Development and Implementation of Clinical Guidelines: report of the Clinical Guidelines Working Group.* Report from General Practice No 26. London: Royal College of General Practitioners, 1996.
12 Eccles MP, Clapp Z, Grimshaw JM, *et al.* North of England evidence-based guideline development project: Methods of guideline development. *BMJ* 1996;312:760–1.
13 Hayward RSA, Wilson MC, Tunis SR, Bass EB, Guyatt G. Users' guides to the medical literature. VII. How to use clinical practice guidelines. A. Are the recommendations valid? *JAMA* 1995;274:570–4.
14 Wilson MC, Hayward RSA, Tunis SR, Bass EB, Guyatt G. Users' guides to the medical literature. VII. How to use clinical practice guidelines. B. What are the recommendations and will they help you in caring for your patients? *JAMA* 1995;274:1630–2.
15 Barratt A, Irwig L, Glasziou P, *et al.* Users' guides to the medical literature: XVII. How to use guidelines and recommendations about screening. Evidence-Based Medicine Working Group. *JAMA* 1999;281:2029–34.
16 Eccles MP, Clapp Z, Grimshaw JM, *et al.* Developing valid guidelines: methodological and procedural issues from the North of England Evidence Based Guideline Development Project. *Qual Health Care* 1996;5:44–50.
17 US Department of Health and Human Services, Public Health Service, Agency for Health Care Policy and Research. *Acute pain management: operative or medical procedures and trauma.* AHCPR Pub 92–0038. Rockville, MD: Agency for Health Care Policy and Research Publications, 1992.
18 North of England Stable Angina Guideline Development Group. North of England evidence-based guideline development project: summary version of evidence-based guideline for primary care management of stable angina. *BMJ* 1996;312:827–31.
19 Lomas J. Teaching old (and not so old) docs new tricks: effective ways to implement research findings. In Dunn EV, Norton PG, Stewart M, Tudiver F, Bass MJ, eds. *Disseminating research/changing practice. Research methods for Primary Care,* vol 6. Thousand Oaks: Sage Publications, 1994.
20 McDonald CJ. Protocol-based computer reminders, the quality of care and the non-perfectability of Man. *N Engl J Med* 1976;295:1351–5.
21 Bero L, Grilli R, Grimshaw JM, Mowatt G, Oxman AD, eds. Cochrane Effective Professional and Organisation of Care Group. In: *Cochrane Collaboration. The Cochrane Library,* Issue 1. Oxford: Update Software, 1999.
22 NHS Centre for Reviews and Dissemination (1999) Getting evidence into

practice. *Effective Health Care Bull* 1999;5:1–16 (also available from: www.york.ac.uk/inst/crd/ehc51.pdf).

23 Mittman BS, Tonesk X, Jacobson PD. Implementing clinical practice guidelines: social influence strategies and practitioner behaviour change. *Qual Rev Bull* 1992;18:413–22.

24 Davis DA, Thomson MA, Oxman AD, Haynes RB. Changing physician performance: a systematic review of the effect of continuing medical education strategies. *JAMA* 1995;274:700–5.

25 Wensing M, Grol R. Single and combined strategies for implementing changes in primary care: a literature review. *Int J Qual Health Care* 1994;6:115–32.

26 Agency for Health Care Policy and Research. *Using clinical guidelines to evaluate quality of care.* vol 1: Issues. AHCPR Pub No. 95–0045. US Department of Health and Human Services, Public Health Service, 1995.

27 Hadorn DC, Baker DW, Kamberg CJ, Brooks RH. Phase II of the AHCPR-sponsored heart failure guideline: translating practice recommendations into review criteria. *Joint Commission Journal Quality Improvement* 1996;22:265–76.

28 Antiplatelet Trialists' Collaboration. Collaborative overview of randomised trials of antiplatelet therapy – I: Prevention of death, myocardial infarction, and stroke by prolonged antiplatelet therapy in various categories of patients. *BMJ* 1994;308:81–106.

10: Role of information technology

MICHAEL KIDD AND IAN PURVES

Introduction

Computers, to a varying degree, have become key tools for every general practice around the world. They have the potential to assist us in management planning, coordination of care, providing continuing medical education and in the process of disseminating research findings. This computer assistance will make us more efficient and effective health care providers if used carefully in the consultation.[1] Information technology has the potential to be the cornerstone of the delivery of evidence-based health care.

This chapter reviews some of the problems associated with attempting to disseminate evidence-based information and examines some of the existing information technology tools that can be used to assist in this process as well as the evidence for their effectiveness. It concludes with a discussion about future developments.

Previous chapters have highlighted the difficulties faced in both accessing and sorting through the large amount of research based information that is available and relevant to our discipline. Even being able to access and keep up to date with summaries of research-based information – whether they be in the form of systematic reviews, clinical practice guidelines, or other distilled, evidence-based recommendations – poses a challenge to primary health care teams worldwide.

The development of the Internet has represented a major advance in terms of facilitating access (both for patients and health professionals) to a wide range of medical information. The quality of some of this information is often questionable. People with no qualification to speak with authority on a topic may do so on the Internet. In the words of Nicholas Negroponte, author of *Being digital*: "On the net, no-one need know you're a dog."[2] The first published systematic survey of health information for the public on the Internet was about managing children with fever at home and found that few of the web pages provided complete and accurate information.[3]

The implications of dissemination of inaccurate research or non-research are far reaching and of significant concern. The day is not too far away when most patients will consult a web based medical site or "electronic doctor" before they come to see a health professional, and possibly to decide whether they need to consult one at all. Already there are some excellent "vetted" lay information sources available on the Internet (for example, Medical Matrix; http://www.medmatrix.org/index.ASP, see Appendix 2). Patients may reconsult these and other information sources after they have seen their health care provider to make sure they have been given the "correct" information and then decide whether to follow the management advice, see another health care provider, or call their lawyer. Throughout this last century, people were consulting home-doctor books; now the volume of information available to patients is many times greater.

Whilst many of the information technology tools currently available can assist users and health professionals in managing the volume of information available, there is also a need for caution in that the technology should not be permitted to dominate our capacity for critical reading and analysis of the information being transmitted. Most of us do not read every line of every medical journal and newspaper that is sent to us. As professionals, we have developed methods of managing this paper based information. We need to develop similar methods to manage electronic information such as e-mail and the Internet.[4]

The information presented to health professionals is usually paper based. When it is needed. we either cannot remember it, never knew it, have no time to access it, or, if we do, cannot find it. We know that general practitioners will use a limited number of readily available resources, such as up-to-date national prescribing "formularies" (for example, *MIMS, British National Formulary*), but our individual information sources are limited during consultations.

Among the advantages of many information technology tools is their capacity to help organise and present complex information in a more structured way than is possible by traditional means of dissemination. They also have the potential to provide real time help in consultations, which overcomes the need for having to spend extra time specifically devoted to tracking down and evaluating information.

Currently available information technology resources

At present, e-mail is becoming increasingly popular among general practitioners and offers us practical benefits already. The advice of experts can be sought electronically. This is particularly advantageous in rural and remote areas, and is already being used as a communication mechanism between primary health care professionals and specialists throughout many parts of the world. E-mail distribution is also being used to relay emergency notifications of pressing health issues from central government to local regions and thence to individual doctors. Advice leaflets for patients can also be included. New guidelines and important research findings are delivered in this way too.

List-servers allow one person to send a single message to all people in the world interested in a particular topic. List-servers like Evidence Based Medicine, GP-UK, Fam-Med and GP-WONCA allow primary health care professionals to collaborate and share information and research findings around the world. The Evidence Based Medicine list-server provides a forum for discussion amongst health care professionals with an interest in evidence-based medicine. Frequently, an individual practitioner will post a clinical problem on the list-server and request assistance from other members about an aspect of how to track down the evidence, evaluate the evidence, or apply the evidence. The list-server also contains information about specialised courses and workshops in evidence-based medicine around the world.

Electronic journals are becoming available, at least in part, on the internet. Electronic versions of the *British Medical Journal, Lancet, Journal of the American Medical Association* and *New England Journal of Medicine* are all available. Several journals are available in full text without subscription. MEDLINE is available free of charge from a number of sites. Directories of clinical information, including research findings, have been created for general practitioners, including the comprehensive Medical Matrix initiative from the USA (http://www.medmatrix.org/index.ASP). Hypertext-based resource materials for medicine, such as the Visible Human Project (http://www.nlm.nih.gov/research/visible/visible_human.html), are available for the education of health professionals and patients. (See Appendix 2.)

A major international development has been the "Clinical Practice Guidelines" initiative of the Agency for Health Care Policy and Research within the Department of Health and Human Services in the USA. This project provides guidelines on line and on CD Rom. It includes a "Quick Reference Guide for Clinicians", with a summary of points for ready reference on a day-to-day basis, and a user version, with information for the general public to increase patient knowledge and involvement in health care decision making. These guidelines include the management of conditions such as acute pain, depression, early HIV infection, heart failure, otitis media in children and benign prostatic hyperplasia. (See Box 9.1 for list of electronic guideline resources.)

Evidence of the effectiveness of information technology in changing practice

In recent years, several major systematic reviews on the use of information technology in information dissemination in medical practice have been carried out. Systematic reviews of the best ways to get clinical guidelines used by doctors[5,6] suggested that they were more likely to be effective if they "take into account local circumstances, are disseminated by an active, educational intervention and implemented by patient-specific reminders". Clearly, information technology provides a means to integrate reminders into the consultation. Bulk mail-outs to doctors and publication in medical journals are far less effective. This was no news to the pharmaceutical industry.

Johnston *et al.* systematically reviewed the effect of computer-based decision support systems on clinician performance and patient outcomes and showed that they can improve clinical performance.[7] Of course, the basis for the information in the computerised decision support systems should come from clinical research. Sullivan and Mitchell also reviewed 21 studies which showed an improvement in clinician performance when a computer was used.[8]

Using these two systematic reviews,[7,8] Table 10.1 shows the differing types of decision support, their level of evaluation in general practice and their effectiveness. The fraction x/y in each cell shows the number of positive studies (x) against the total number of studies performed (y). Although the evidence is limited, it suggests that computerised decision support is more likely to be effective for management decisions than for diagnosis. More recent evaluations also support these findings.[9-13] Simple prompting and reminder systems have been more extensively evaluated, with consistently positive results, than knowledge based and other more "advanced" systems.

Table 10.1 Types of decision support and their effectiveness

Type of computerised system	GP process	GP outcomes	All Process	All outcomes
Differential diagnosis	–	–	1/5	1/1
Drug dose calculation	–	–	3/4	0/3
Reminder	6/6	–	8/9	0/1
Alert	–	–	1/1	–
Protocol	4/5	1/1	7/8	1/3

The future

Predicting the nature and extent of information technology solutions likely to be available in the 21st century is fraught with danger. However, there are a number of possible scenarios. For example, it is likely that "electronic clearing houses" will be developed to assist the dissemination of research findings for primary care. This is a role which may be taken on by individuals, and by regional and national professional, primary care organisations as a service to members or by university-based groups. It is also possible that commercial groups will take on this role as a means of advertising and supporting the profession.

It will not be long before the majority of us have instant access to the Internet in our consulting rooms. In Canada, pharmacies are already connected to a health intranet and so receive instant feedback on their' dispensing. In Australia, the General Practice National Information Service Internet site (http://som.flinders.edu.au/FUSA/GPNIS/Default.html) provides information on completed general practice research projects in Australia, an electronic newsletter, the facility for e-mail discussion groups on research topics, lists of publications and support materials and information on conferences. Services like this will expand and develop and become more interactive as the technology develops.

Electronic medication management provides a practical example of developing information technology which many general practitioners have adopted over the past 12 months. In the UK, over 70% of doctors prescribe with electronic prescriptions (over 90% for repeats) and over 80% of doctors use a computer in the consultation. This allows doctors rapid access to information about medications (i.e. the results of research findings) as well as the decision support features of cross-checking for contraindications, adverse reactions and allergy alerts. It also offers the benefits of improved legibility, accuracy and recording of prescription data. This use of computerised decision support has the potential to be the most significant benefit of information technology towards improving the quality of general practice.[14,15]

One logical extension of evidence-based practice is that research findings will be utilised to develop guidelines for clinical management. One example of such a project (known as the Prodigy Project[16,17]) is currently being evaluated in the UK. The project incorporates guidelines developed by national bodies for use in general practice as part of seven different computerised medical record systems which are available to general practitioners. At this stage, very few of the guidelines are evidence-based. The general practitioner types in the diagnosis, picks a code and guidelines for management and prescribing for that condition appear. This information may be viewed by the patient on the screen or may be printed out. Also, as the Prodigy guidelines can interact with existing electronic medication management systems, they can prompt about possible contraindications, adverse reactions and known drug allergies.

Whilst it is important that efforts are made to ensure that guidelines promoted by systems such as Prodigy are evidence-based, there is also the potential to explore how guidelines might be personalised for individual patients and made more interactive with additional decision support features.

It is inevitable as we now enter the next millennium that the nature of general practice will change. Early solutions to the problems of dissemination do exist and are in use. However, underlying these developments we must preserve the doctor–patient relationship. At the same time we cannot ignore doctors' need for information; and we need to develop effective ways of dealing with patients who present with detailed, evidence-based, medical information. In the Information Age, should we keep ahead of our patients or should we work together, share the information and develop management plans together? We face many big challenges. Although the doctor–patient interaction will remain the major focus of our work, increasingly both doctor and patient will be utilising and relying on information technology and electronic connections to the rest of the world through which the dissemination of research findings will occur.

References

1 Purves IN. Facing future challenges in general practice: a clinical method with computer support. *Fam Pract* 1996;13:536–43.
2 Negroponte N. *Being digital.* New York: Alfred A Knopf, 1995.
3 Impicciatore P, Pandolfini C, Casella N, Bonati M. Information in practice. Reliability of health information for the public on the World Wide Web: systematic survey of advice on managing fever in children at home. *BMJ* 1997;314:1879–81.
4 Purves IN, Bainbridge M, Trimble I. Running a medical mailing list. In: McKenzie BC, ed. *Medicine and the Internet.* Oxford: Oxford University Press, 1997.
5 Grimshaw JM, Russell IT. Effect of clinical guidelines on medical practice: a systematic review of rigorous evaluations. *Lancet* 1993;342:1317–22.
6 Grimshaw JM, Russell IT. Implementing clinical practice guidelines: can guidelines be used to improve clinical practice? *Effective Health Bull* 1994;8.
7 Johnston ME, Langton KB, Haynes KB, Mathieu A. The effects of computer-based clinical decision support systems on clinician performance and patient outcomes. A critical appraisal of research. *Ann Intern Med* 1994;120:135–42.
8 Sullivan F, Mitchell E. Has general practitioner computing made a difference to patient care? A systematic review of published reports. *BMJ* 1995;311:848–52.
9 Balas EA, Austin SM, Mitchell JA, Ewigman BG, Bopp KD, Brown GD. The clinical value of computerized information services: a review of 98 randomized clinical trials. *Arch Fam Med* 1996;5:271–78.
10 Pestonik SL, Classen DC, Scott Evans R, Burke JP. Implementing antibiotic practice guidelines through computer-assisted decision support: clinical and financial outcomes. *Ann Intern Med* 1996;124:884–90.
11 Beilby JJ, Silagy CA. Trials of providing costing information to general practitioners: a systematic review. *Med J Aust* 1997;167:89–92.
12 Hunt DL, Haynes RB, Hanna SE, Smith K. Effects of computer-based clinical decision support systems on physician performance and patient outcomes – a systematic review. *JAMA* 1998;280:1339–46.
13 Young JM, Ward JE. General practitioners' use of evidence databases. *Med J Aust* 1999;170:56–8.

14 Department of Human Services and Health and IBM Consulting Group. *Electronic prescribing and medicine information consultancy*. Canberra: IBM Consultancy Group, 1996.
15 Frank O, Kidd MR. A guide to computer-generated prescriptions. *Aust Fam Phys* 1996;7:1162–63.
16 Purves IN, Sowerby M. Prodigy interim report. *J Informatics Primary Care* 1996; (Sept): 2–8.
17 Purves IN, Sowerby M, Beaumont R, Sugden R. An aristocrat, a precocious child, and a sacred cow. Developing general practice clinical computer systems: a collaboration between general practitioners, system suppliers and the NHS Executive – lessons from the Prodigy methodology. In: *Proceedings of the Annual Conference of the Primary Health Care Steering Group of the British Computer Society*,1996;51–73.

11: Continuing medical education as a means of lifelong learning

DAVE DAVIS AND MARY ANN O'BRIEN

Objectives and overview

This chapter builds upon the professional behaviour change strategies, first introduced in Chapter 8, by exploring how health care professionals can incorporate an evidence-based approach into their own lifelong learning and continuing education.

First, we explore how professionals learn. We have developed a series of case scenarios to highlight the importance of using needs assessment and available evidence of effectiveness to tailor choices of educational methods and opportunities to the clinical capability to be addressed. Throughout, we introduce examples and ideas of how general practitioners can apply the principles of evidence-based health care as part of their practice.

Theories of adult learning

Origins

Numerous theories of learning have been developed, some applying mostly or exclusively to adults. In order to make sense of the huge body of literature, a number of classifications have been proposed, with Saddington's "five traditions" being among the most useful.[1] Each tradition is underpinned by a particular ideological and philosophical stance and is characterised by different overall goals, views of the educator, the learner and his or her experience. The two traditions most frequently associated with continuing medical education (CME) are the technological (or behavioural) and the humanistic.

The technological tradition aims to improve performance, production and efficiency based on pre-set observable, measurable and behavioural objectives. The educator's role is to instruct, and the educated person is described as competent. The learner's experience determines the point of entry to the learning process but is otherwise not central. It is probably easy for doctors to recognise this approach to CME. However, it originates from the work of behavioural psychologists, such as Skinner,[2] and as such has connotations of social control.

In the humanistic tradition, personal development and growth are the goals. The educator's task is to support the learner or facilitate interaction between learners and the educated person is "integrated" or person-centred. The learner's own experience is used as a source of knowledge and to shape the curriculum. It is likely once again that you recognise this model – it has strongly influenced GP vocational training in the UK and has its roots in the work of Rogers, Knowles, and Schon.[1,3-5] It is linked to notions of autonomy and freedom and the development of self-directed learning.

This field is fraught with terminological difficulties.[6] For example, the terms "competence" and "competency" have slightly different meanings in the UK, North America and Australia, all to a greater or lesser extent allied to the technological tradition of adult learning.[7,8] Professional competence is often broken down into lists of specific competences[9] or competencies.[10] Here we have used *competence* only to refer to observable or measurable phenomena. We have used the term "capability" as a catch-all term for what we do as it is relatively free from association with any one tradition, ideology or mode of learning.

Performance causes less confusion and refers to the actual activities of the professional in the *real* work setting. It is important to note that competence in a simulated or test environment is not always the same as true performance.[11]

Gaps in professional practice are sometimes split into three domains: knowledge, skills and attitudes. We recognise the separation is artificial (it is usually impossible to tease out why we do what we do in the way that we do) but it is sometimes helpful to consider these domains independently.

Relevance to continuing medical education for general practice

The learner-centred ethos of the humanistic tradition is likely to have face validity for general practitioners and clear resonance with patient-centred approaches in clinical practice. The tenets of holism and respect for the individual and their experience suggest shared values and attitudes between these two approaches.

To the adult his (sic) experience is him. He defines who he is, establishes his self identity, in terms of a unique series of experiences...he has a deep investment in the value of his experience. And so, when he finds himself in a situation in which his experience is not used, or its worth is minimized, it is not just his experience that is being rejected.[4]

However, it is important to take the parallel further and acknowledge that a major limitation of the learner-centred approach is the difficulty in distinguishing educational "wants" from "needs". The technological tradition relies on attempts to identify deficiencies using actual or proxy measures of clinical performance or outcome. What emerges is the need for a model that incorporates the learner-centred processes of the humanistic approach balanced by a concern for appropriate clinical goals.

Common themes

Recently, models of adult learning have been developed which help to draw together different theories.[7,10,12] Common themes emerge, resulting in a more integrated and holistic overall approach to continuing professional education while stressing the need to tailor specific methods to particular goals. The four common themes are:

(1) learner motivation
(2) assessing learning needs and professional gaps
(3) enhancing reflection
(4) developing a personal framework for relating theory to practice (or in the specific case of evidence-based health care, relating evidence to experience) in order to change and move on.

The practical relevance of these themes is illustrated by the example shown in Box 11.1. Dr Sheila Robertson's problem (Box 11.1) is not uncommon; many general practitioners experience changing demands during their career. It raises several important questions which are central to understanding adult learning. Firstly, what factors have influenced Sheila's decision to return to primary care practice (motivation)? Secondly, what are the gaps between Sheila's current and desired capabilities, and how should these be identified (needs assessment and reflection)? Thirdly, what resources and strategies are available to assist Sheila in meeting her learning needs (learning style and opportunities)? How relevant and effective are they (relating experience to evidence base)?

Box 11.1   Case study 1

Sheila Robertson completed a general practice training programme in the UK 7 years ago. Busy with family commitments since then, she has maintained her clinical capabilities in two ways: first, she has worked in a unit for the elderly one day per week; second, she has attended regular CME events, particularly in health care of the elderly, but in other areas as well. She is now returning to general practice and is anxious about looking after a mixed population, including children, once again. What can she do to improve and to assure herself of her clinical capabilites?

It is likely that Sheila is well motivated (an internal factor) to make the change to taking on full practice responsibilities since she has already shown a willingness and commitment to trying to keep up to date. In addition, Sheila is relatively young, a factor which has been demonstrated as a significant predictor of professional competence.[13] Part of the change process for Sheila will need to include an assessment of her current knowledge and skills compared to those required when she returns to full-time practice.[14,15] These will be discussed further below. Once the nature of any gap between her ideal and actual competence has been defined, Sheila will need to make a plan for learning that is both manageable, and achievable. For example, it may be that she will need to begin by reviewing the demographics of her new practice to determine the kinds of patient problems that are high volume, high risk or high cost.[16] In a young, healthy population, it may be that her major learning needs are for the provision of immunisation and preventive care.

The evidence base

The evaluation of the theories described and the educational strategies derived from them tend to use the qualitative methods of sociology, psychology and anthropology. Nonetheless, where quantitative and systematic evidence of effectiveness of the different educational approaches does exist,[17] the results tend to support the need for a holistic approach to CME which incorporates prior needs assessment, interaction and personal focus while keeping clear goals in mind. As with patient-centred medicine, learner-centred education started out as a value-driven ideal and is now being shown to contribute to measurable improvements in professional capability.

Needs assessment: identifying gaps in professional capability

One of the key challenges that health professionals face is knowing whether or not their current practice is up to date. Sackett and colleagues[18] refer to this as "the key to continued effectiveness as a clinician." The range of different needs assessment techniques (adapted from Dixon, 1978)[19] can be summarised as a continuum (Box 11.2).

At the left-hand end of the continuum are perceived needs, which are usually assessed using subjective methods based on personal reflection.[5,7,20–23] When using such methods, the responsibility for recognising gaps in a given clinical situation, and for choosing and using appropriate learning resources to address them, rests squarely with the health professional, perhaps with the guidance of a mentor.[24]

Although there are a wide variety of ways in which health professionals,' can develop the capacity to subjectively assess their own learning needs, they all have a common theme: comparing what we do (as health professionals) to what our colleagues do, to what our patients or funders expect, or to what the evidence suggests we should be doing.

Box 11.2   Needs assessment techniques

	SUBJECTIVE	OBJECTIVE	
Self	*Competence*	*Performance*	*Patient outcomes*

• Reflection on:
 – patient
   encounter
 – significant
   event
 – reading
 – course
   attended
 – discussion
   with peers
 – self-audit/log
	• Multiple choice
	   quizzes (knowledge)
	 • Objective structured
	   clinical examinations
	   (clinical skills/
	   method)
	 • Simulated
	   consultations
		• Simulated patient
		   in real practice
		 • Chart review
		 • External audit with
		   feedback (for
		   example, use of
		   diagnostics, drugs)
		 • Targets (for example
		   immunisations,
		   cytology
			• Clinical review

While some health professionals would argue that they can easily identify and understand their own learning needs, there is evidence that we may benefit most from studying topics that we do not select and that we tend to select topics we already know quite well.[25,26]

On reflection

If the "key to continued clinical effectiveness" is keeping up to date then it could be argued that the key to keeping up to date is the enhancement of reflection. Although all the referenced authors take a slightly different view, the unifying principle is the capability to return to and re-evaluate an experience (an encounter with a real patient, simulated patient or a paper case; a personal life-event, activities on a course; or reading a journal) in order to identify professional gaps and make sense of how their own frameworks for understanding knowledge and practice fit together and can be altered. Although definitive evidence to support these ideas is lacking, results from medical graduates of problem-based curricula suggest that they have enhanced reflective capabilities and undertake more self-directed learning once qualified.[27] In the absence of compelling research evidence, the accumulated view of the importance of reflection in continuing professional education by every author in the field is difficult to ignore.

Several tools exist to help combine reflective or subjective needs assessment methods with use of objective methods, such as measures of competence (for example, objective, structured clinical examinations), performance (for example, external audits), patient management problems and health outcomes (Box 11.2).[28–31] Each of these strategies may be helpful in identifying unrecognised learning needs and assessment measures for knowledge, skills and attitudes. Performance measures are then used to assess what happens in real practice.

Patient encounters frequently provoke an awareness of an educational need – an unusual presentation, a missed diagnosis, an unexpected death, a patient complaint or a bureaucratic mishap (such as a lost test result) are all examples of significant events that may indicate new or refreshed capabilities are required. Dr Margit Petersen's story (Box 11.3) highlights how the process of reflection can be triggered by a conflict between our practice and that indicated by the evidence.

Box 11.3   Case study 2

Margit Petersen is a 35-year-old general practitioner in Ontario, treating an uncomplicated 50-year-old person with hypertension. After the suggested three-visit recording of his blood pressure, and determining that it is regularly over 160/105, she starts him on an angiotensin-converting enzyme inhibitor and is fairly happy with her results: on the next two visits it is 140/95 and 138/92. She is fairly happy, that is, until she attends a small-group CME session at which she learns that many of her colleagues abide by the current national preventive guidelines which recommend a diuretic and/or beta-blocker as first-line therapy.

Many health professionals develop a regular process of scanning journals, reading course brochures, reviewing consultation letters, reading other doctors' notes in the group practice, and discussing specific cases with peers.

Review or audit of medical records (see Chapter 7) is a useful method of determining the extent to which our current practice is consistent with evidence-based principles. The example shown in Box 11.4 illustrates one approach.

The selection of all records in a particular age category (like Dr Peter O'Hanion's case in Box 11.4) or other risk categories (for example, women in the case of breast or cervical screening guidelines) is especially useful when looking for compliance with screening guidelines. Other methods include use of random record audit, or a day book to identify patient

---

Box 11.4   Case study 3

Peter O'Hanion has read the recent guidelines on flu vaccine for geriatric patients and for those with certain other conditions. He believes that he and his partner do pretty well in the 65-and-over age category, but his partner is not quite so optimistic. Peter says they have 90% compliance with the guidelines and that the 10% of patients who do not comply are those whom they cannot reach by phone or who flatly refuse the injection. To prove a point, he asks his nurse to pull all the medical records of patients over 65 (not a difficult task given the relatively small number involved, and a new computer system which allows them to retrieve chart numbers by disease or demographic variables). In Peter's case, only 55% of his geriatric patients received annual flu injections.

---

records for study and review. In other instances. information may be fed back to health professionals from government or private health insurance groups with information about our service utilisation that allows comparison of our "score" to other more global data (for example, the number of antibiotics prescribed per patient against an average for all similar physicians).

Continuing education choices – making the most of the opportunities

Having identified learning needs through a combination of measures, the next step is to select appropriate continuing education opportunities. The range of opportunities that exists is almost endless (from conferences to peer consultations, self-assessment programmes to use of standardised patients). The challenge is to try to categorise these learning resources in a way which enables comparisons to be made regarding their effectiveness (Table 11.1).[17] A taxonomy that has been used elsewhere includes traditional methods such as *educational materials* (printed, audio, or videotapes) and conferences (courses, symposia and rounds) as well as more innovative methods (such as use of opinion leaders, academic detailing and patient-mediated interventions). The more traditional methods have been shown in controlled trials to result in minimal change in practitioner performance compared with the more innovative methods. However, the traditional methods may assist in predisposing health professionals to change by fostering prerequisite attitudes or increasing specific areas of knowledge or skills. The more interactive the traditional methods are (for example, use of hands-on workshops), the more likely they are to result in changes in performance.[17]

Table 11.1 Effectiveness of learning resources on fulfilment of learning needs

	Knowledge	Attitudes	Skills	Performance
Educational materials	+	?	?	–
Didactic conferences	+	?	–	–
Courses with interaction	+	+/–	+	+/–
Opinion leaders	+	+	?	+
Outreach (detailing)	+	?	?	+
Local consensus process	+	+	?	–
Patient-mediated strategies	?	?	–	+
Audit and feedback	+	+	?	+/–
Marketing	+	+	?	+
Reminders	?	?	?	+

+ = improvement based on evidence from randomised controlled trials
? = evidence is unclear or unavailable
– = no improvement based on evidence from randomised controlled trials

The practical implementation of different CME opportunities and strategies is illustrated in the three case studies shown in Boxes 11.5, 11.9 and 11.11.

Dr Ashish Bhageria (Box 11.5) represents a growing group of general practitioners who actively pay attention to their learning needs through structured reflection. Unlike most of us, they were trained in an undergraduate environment which made explicit those components of learning such as needs assessment, accessing resources, self-evaluation, and knowing your preferred personal learning style. Even more importantly, they gave permission to the learner to say: "I don't know the answer to that question, but I can find out."[27]

Box 11.5   Case study 4

Ashish Bhageria is a 32-year-old physician who recently completed an Australian general practice training programme, and, perhaps more importantly, is a graduate of a problem-based undergraduate curriculum. He has kept a "learning log", a holdover from his undergraduate days, and a tool which has maintained his competence over his 3 years in practice.

At the end of the day, the log displays two remaining questions from the day's practice: one related to the interaction of two medications (an anticonvulsant and an antibiotic) and one related to the more complicated issue of managing the menopause.

A wide array of learning resources is available to clinicians such as Dr Bhageria who wish to acquire knowledge about specific subjects or areas. Box 11.6 groups these resources according to the degree to which they are likely to be evidence-based.[17]

Ashish determines that it is his learning style which will ultimately direct his choice of resources to meet his learning needs: he is a voracious reader, and has developed a pattern of communication with peers and specialists

---

Box 11.6   Types of learning resources characterised by the degree they are most often based on evidence[17]

Potential for evidence based practice

Low	Medium	High
• Pharmaceutical monographs	• Medical school conferences	• Academic detailing/ outreach
• Pharmaceutical sales representatives	• Meetings of scientific/ scholarly organisations	• Evidence-based journals
• "CME" dinners (drug company sponsored)	• Consensus conference guidelines	• Evidence-based guidelines
	• Texts (depending on sponsor)	
	• Most peer-reviewed journals	
	• Video/audiotapes (depending on sponsor)	

---

that permits him to feel comfortable in formal CME. And so, before leaving for home that evening, he undertakes two CME activities. First, he does a brief review of the drug interaction question in his drugs and therapeutics reference book, which lists most common medications by brand and chemical name, their methods of action, side effects and interactions. Such books go by a variety of names and although they are not always based on systematic reviews of the research, they do indicate specific interactions and cautions. In this case, the book suggests that patients' anticonvulsant blood levels should be monitored during concurrent treatment. Telephoning his patient to make this arrangement, Ashish also notes this question for further literature searching.

Using the literature

When, for example through reading, peer discussion, or attending a course, we encounter an instance where our current practice is at odds with that of others, the major questions to address are as follows:

- Is there a broad general area about which I do not know much or have a learning need?
- How does my approach compare with the one I have just heard or read about?
- What is the evidence that this other practice is better (or based on better evidence) than my current one?
- What do I need to change in order to bring my practice in line with the desired practice?
- How can I incorporate this change in my practice?

Sackett and colleagues[18] have developed an approach to the potentially laborious task of journal reading for busy practitioners. (Box 11.7).

Box 11.7 Scanning the medical literature (or any other source of medical information)[18]

Step 1: am I receiving the correct medical journals (CME flyers, monographs, newsletters)?

Step 2: do I set aside time to regularly read the title page on a relatively timely basis?

Step 3: do the titles/subjects look interesting and relevant?

Step 4: if so, does the abstract/summary/objectives look useful to me (given that the findings are valid, of course)?

Step 5: is the setting of the study (review article, CME topic) similar to mine?

Step 6: could I apply this information (for example, diagnosis, treatment, causation, prognosis) in practice?

The second question for Ashish is harder to answer. He has encountered several women in his practice recently with menopausal symptoms, and he starts wondering about how best to manage them. Although he is quite knowledgeable about the dosing of oestrogen and the need for use of progesterone, he is uncertain about a number of questions such as the risk of breast cancer and osteoporosis. He elects to find a course to attend in the next several months which will address these questions.

Box 11.8 Choosing your learning activities: some criteria for the selection of CME courses* with potential for impact on practice

Step 1: relevance
- Is the theme of the course* relevant to my practice and my educational needs?
- Are there specific objectives (for example, "at the conclusion of this conference the participant will be able to develop a disease-prevention routine for postmenopausal women on HRT")?
- Do these objectives match my practice, patients and own needs?

Step 2: credibility
- Who is the major sponsor of the activity?
- Is it a credible body (for example, a professional association or medical school)?
- If credible, does the activity have significant support from a potentially biased source (for example, industry support may be mentioned on the course brochure, may have reduced registration costs considerably, or added benefits to the course not usually acceptable, such as free social activities)?
- Does the phrase "evidence based" or "a review of the literature" appear in workshop or lecture titles?

Step 3: format
- Does the format allow *interactivity*, (for example, a scheduled question and answer session or the use of audience response systems)?
- Is there a balance between formal lectures/didactic talks and workshops where patient and other practical problems can be addressed?
- Are there small-group sessions?
- Is there an attempt to provide ongoing learning resources (for example, printed materials such as a course syllabus, references, electronic mail or other means) to extend the learning beyond the programme?

Step 4: logistics
- Is the conference location convenient?
- Is the venue comfortable and suitable for learning?

---

* "Course" is a broad term used here to encompass all formal CME activities described as conferences, symposia, meetings, workshops

---

Choosing courses

Choosing a CME course deserves careful consideration. Not all courses or conferences are of equal value. Furthermore, participating in a conference

– regardless of its quality – may or may not result in practice changes or knowledge gain. Nonetheless, the evidence about conferences and courses indicates that the most successful are those which follow the principles (outlined in Box 11.8) of choice by relevance and applicability; credibility; opportunity for discussion, feedback and practice integration; and logistics.

Box 11.9 Case study 5

The Mayo Foundation has just established a new primary care clinic in rural Minnesota, and has asked Joao Nunes to become a teacher-practitioner in the community, responsible for training two trainees per year. Joao, who has been an active, "big city" doctor with the Mayo system for over 10 years, wants to do this, but says to the head of the training programme: "I'm apprehensive about the move: for one thing, I haven't done obstetrics in 5 years, and for another, I'm not so sure about my teaching skills." He goes on to explain his fears about his level of knowledge and capability to teach residents and this "evidence based thing". What advice would you give him if you were the head of the training programme?

In answer to the question posed in Case study 5 (Box 11.9), fortunately, the head of the training programme, following the process outlined in this chapter, can summarise for Joao the differences in the kinds of skills which

---

Box 11.10 Skills in primary care and general practice: types, examples and learning methods

Type of skill	Examples	Learning resources
Manual	Obstetrics	Traineeship
	Suturing	Apprenticing
Communication	Interviewing	Specially designed courses*
	Counselling	Traineeships
Office management	Record keeping	Courses*
		Working with colleagues/apprenticeship, small groups, employing chart review
		Computers
		Courses*
		Training with computer "experts"
		Practice
Evidence based	Journal reading, searching	Courses*
medicine	Appraising the literature	Small groups
	Applying the evidence	Apprenticing
		Reading and practice
Teaching	Small-group facilitation	Peer mentoring, consultations
	One-to-one supervision	Peer/faculty development groups
	Planning presentations, teaching sessions and courses	Courses*
		Reading
	Critiquing performance and providing feedback	Peer observation, quality circle, audio/videotape

* Always look for courses that permit training opportunities for rehearsal with simulations (for example, suturing labs or role-playing with standardised patients) and the opportunity for feedback on learning

---

his new move will require and the range of learning options which can be utilised (Box 11.10). In Joao's case, the need to upgrade skills in obstetrics would probably require a clinical "traineeship" in the form of a one- to several week-long training experience which provides an opportunity for real patient care under supervised circumstances. Apprenticeships or joining a colleague for deliveries may be an acceptable, if less structured alternative. In the case of Joao's need to improve his teaching skills, especially in critical appraisal, many options are open to him – small groups, peer mentoring, reading, and consultations are all viable options. We should note that, if acquiring new skills or upgrading old ones is the objective, the use of simulations (for example, mannikins in the case of cardiac resuscitation courses, standardised patients and/or role playing in communication or counselling skills courses) is a necessary ingredient.

Challenging attitudes

While Dr McCrimmon (Box 11.11) may be an extreme example of an "attitude" problem, we all suffer from deficits in our practice in relation to our values and beliefs. There are two useful ways to characterise these attitudes, described as attitudes "to" and attitudes "about" issues. Under the "to" category, we might ask ourselves whether our attitudes to certain patients carry judgemental elements, for example to patients of different sexual orientations or ethnocultural backgrounds, especially when these characteristics are different than our own. Further, attitudes to others may include peers, specialists, government or other regulatory bodies and – in some ways most importantly – to ourselves. Attitudes "about issues" are similarly of a wide variety including patient personal choice such as abortion or lifestyle and other, more regulatory or practice-controlling issues like managed care.[32]

Box 11.11 Case study 6

Dr Dunc McCrimmon is a 55-year-old general practitioner from California, who has been called to the local regulatory body because of a complaint lodged by the family of Jose Ramirez, a 42-year-old, long-term patient of Dunc's. Mr Ramirez presented to his doctor's office, complaining of severe insomnia and worry about excess drinking, and was prescribed a large supply of chlormethiazole capsules. Having collected the prescription, Jose went home, took an overdose, and was found dead by his family, who subsequently lodged legal and professional action against Dr McCrimmon. When called before the panel, Dr McCrimmon said: "I'm not so sure what the problem is here. Most of these people are too lazy to work, and just want a form filled out or a prescription." On questioning, it became apparent that Dunc did not assess depression nor the potential for suicide in this case, and did not appear to know that prescribing chlormethiazole is, for the most part, contraindicated in instances like this.

Acknowledging problems arising from values and attitudes is far from easy. Often, sadly, they are only exposed by a conflict with a patient or colleagues or, as in this case, by a formal complaint.

Several useful learning resources and formats which might accelerate attitude shifts include small groups that permit considerable peer interaction, frank discussion and even confrontation, traineeships which require (re)learning skills and a certain degree of flexibility and critical examination of one's practice based on others', and practice reflection exercises.[5]

Conclusion – translating learning into practice

There is an old cartoon, depicting an elderly male physician interviewing his young woman patient. "How come you're always here?" she asks. "Don't you believe in CME?" He replies, "Oh, Mrs. Brown, I could go off to courses and such, but I already know more than I practise!" There is considerable truth in the exchange. While all of us are human, most of us have considerable room for improvement, which is possible to achieve (Box 11.12).

Box 11.12 Case study 7

Peter O'Hanion and his partner (whom we met first when discussing performance assessment as a means to discovering learning and practice needs) have decided to correct their "abysmal" (Peter's words) and surprisingly low flu injection rate. This year, they have decided to put into place a four part programme, no single element of which was very expensive in time or money. They have:

(1) scheduled a regular, noon-hour "flu-shot clinic" for drop-ins, over 4 weeks

(2) put up a large poster supplied by the public health department in the waiting room, reminding patients (and the staff) of the impending flu season

(3) asked reception staff to place yellow "stickies", i.e. reminders, on the front of charts of eligible patients when those patients present for routine or episodic visits

(4) offered a telephone reminder to their non-attenders (done by the office staff).

The final scenario (Box 11.12) highlights several features of the primary care team: they have been able to successfully incorporate the principles of concurrent quality improvement, or total quality management,[16] and thus translate evidence-based education and management into the practice setting. This achievement involves four steps, which also serve as a summary of how to embark on a process of lifelong learning in relation to the practice of evidence-based health care.

The first and perhaps most essential ingredient is the consideration of ourselves as learners, not just practitioners.[24] This involves thinking about our preferred methods of learning, our motivations to change, our age or stage of development, and (even) our attitudes about learning and practising evidence-based health care. The second step is to find ways of determining the gaps between what we do and optimal or desirable practices. The third step incorporates the use of a wide array of learning resources from which we must select those that are most effective for us based on both clinical and educational evidence, and most relevant to the particular facet of knowledge, attitude, or skill we require. The fourth and final step, which is highlighted in the last scenario, relates to considering the practice setting as a comprehensive team involving patients, a range of health professionals and support staff, all of whom need to work together in an ongoing partnership in order to achieve successful implementation of evidence-based practice.

Acknowledgements

We would like to thank Ms Anne Taylor-Vaisey and Ms Susan Wicks at the University of Toronto for their assistance with the preparation of this chapter.

References

1 Saddington JA. Learner experience: a rich resource for learning. In: Mulligan J, Griffin C, eds. *Empowerment through experiential learning*. London: Kogan Page, 1992, pp 37–49.

2 Skinner BE. *The technology of teaching*. New York, NY: Prentice Hall, 1968.

3 Rogers C. *Freedom to learn for the 80s*. Ohio: Merrill, 1983.

4 Knowles M. *The modern practice of adult education: andragogy and pedagogy*. Chicago: Follet, 1970.

5 Schan DA. *Educating the reflective practitioner: toward a new design for teaching and learning in the professions*. San Francisco, CA: Jossey-Bass, 1990.

6 Barnett R. *The limits of competence*. Buckingham: Open University Press, 1994.

7 Brookfield S. The epistemology of adult education in the US and Great Britain: a cross-cultural analysis. In: Bright B, ed. *Theory and practice in the study of adult education – the epistemological debate*. London: Routledge, 1989.

8 Eraut M. *Developing professional knowledge and competence*. London: Falmer, 1994.

9 Bines H, Watson D. *Developing professional education*. Buckingham: Open University Press, 1992.

10 Jarvis P. *Adult and continuing education: theory and practice*. London: Routledge, 1995.

11 Rethans JJ, Westin S, Hays R. Methods for quality assessment in general practice. *Fam Pract* 1996;13:468–76.

12 Boud D, Cohen R, Walker D. *Using experience for learning*. Buckingham: Open University Press, 1993.

13 Ferrier BM, Woodward CA, Cohen M, Williams AP. Clinical practice guidelines. New-to-practice family physicians' attitudes. *Can Fam Physician* 1996;42:463–8.

14 Fox RD, Mazmanian PE, Putnam RW. *Changing and learning in the lives of physicians*. New York, NY: Praeger Publications, 1989.

15 Bandura A. *Social foundations of thought and action: a social cognitive theory.* Englewood Cliffs, NJ: Prentice-Hall, 1986.

16 Berwick DM. Sounding board – continuous improvement as an ideal in health care. *N Engl J Med* 1989;320:53–6.

17 Davis DA, Thomson MIA, Oxman AD, Haynes RB. Changing physician performance: a systematic review of the effect of continuing medical education strategies. *JAMA* 1995;274:700–5.

18 Sackett DL, Haynes RB, Tugwell P. *Clinical epidemiology. A basic science for clinical medicine.* Boston, MA: Little, Brown, 1985.

19 Dixon J. Evaluation criteria in studies of continuing education in the health professions: a critical review of a suggested strategy. *Evaluation Health Professions* 1978;1:47–65.

20 Boud D, Keogh R, Walker D, eds. *Reflection – turning experience into learning.* London: Kogan Page, 1985.

21 Agyris C. *Reasoning, learning, and action.* San Francisco, CA: Jossey Bass Publishers, 1982.

22 Kolb DA. The process of experiential learning. In: Thorpe M, Edwards R, Hanson A, eds. *Culture and process in adult learning: a reader.* London: Routledge/Open University Press, 1993.

23 Freire P. *Pedagogy of the oppressed* (trans. Ramer MB). Harmondsworth: Penguin, 1972.

24 Pietroni R, Mullard L. Portfolio-based learning. In: Pendleton D, Hasler J, eds. *Professional development in general practice.* Oxford: Oxford University Press, 1997.

25 Sibley JC, Sackett DL, Neufeld VR, *et al.* A randomised trial of continuing medical education. *N Engl J Med* 1982;306:511–15.

26 Davis D, O'Brien MA, Freemantle N, Wolf FM, Mazmanian P. Impact of formal continuing medical education: do conferences, workshops, rounds and other traditional continuing education activities change physical behaviour or health care outcomes? *JAMA* 1999; 282:867–74.

27 Norman G, Schmidt H. The psychological basis of problem-based learning: a review of the evidence. *Acad Med* 1992;67:557–65.

28 Neufeld VR, Norman GR, eds. *Assessing clinical competence.* New York, NY: Springer Publishing, 1985.

29 Harden RM, Gleeson FA. Assessment of clinical competence using an objective structured clinical examination (OSCE). *Med Educ* 1979;13:41–54.

30 Craig JL. The OSCME (Opportunity for Self-Assessment CME). *J Contin Educ Health Prof* 1991;11:87–94.

31 Marquis Y, Chaoulli J, Bordage G, Chabot JM, Leclere H. Patient managment problems as a learning tool for the continuing medical education of general practitioners. *Med Educ* 1984;18:117–24.

32 David DA, Fox RD, eds. *The physician as learner: linking research to practice.* Chicago, IL: American Medical Association, 1996.

12: Integrating research evidence into practice

ANDREW HAINES AND STEPHEN ROGERS

Introduction

Culture has been described as "that complex whole which includes knowledge, belief, art, morals, law, custom and any other capabilities and habits".[1]

The five-step process by which evidence-based medicine is practised in relation to individual doctor–patient consultations is developed from the application of epidemiological methods to clinical problems.[2] The approach originated at McMaster University, Ontario, Canada where it has been applied particularly to the management of individual patients. However, application of new clinical knowledge will frequently require changes in the organisation and delivery of services. While evidence-based medicine is the "conscientious, explicit and judicious use of current, best evidence in making decisions about the care of individual patients", with its own information sources, assumptions and techniques, evidence-based practice will require further "capabilities and habits" in order to translate new knowledge into improvements in service. A culture of evidence-based practice would include both the application of best evidence to clinical problem solving and effective implementation of new services to benefit groups of patients.

While various elements of the evidence-based practice approach are represented in primary care, there are conceptual and practical barriers to be overcome before a culture of evidence-based practice will become established.

Integrating art and science in general practice

General practice has always exhibited pluralism in its approach to the complexities of dealing with illness and disease. A culture of evidence-based practice will need to be set in the context of other theoretical and belief systems which characterise general practice.[3] These include not only

157

the biomedical system of hospital medicine, but also the hermeneutic (interpretive) approach,[4] "patient-centred care",[5] anticipatory care, population-based primary care[6] and community-oriented primary care.[7] It will also need to take into account the changing roles of general practitioners, such as their increasing contribution to the planning and commissioning of services through primary care groups and primary care trusts in the UK.

Many factors impinge on general practice such as the beliefs of patients about the cause and appropriate treatment of their condition,[8] family influences on behaviour, socio-economic factors and the pronouncements of policy makers. This is also the case in hospital medicine, though general practitioners may be more aware than most of the modulating effects of patient choice and circumstances, co-morbidity and the constraints imposed by an overstretched health service on whether recommendations resulting from clinical trials and other types of research can be applied with patients. Initiatives that fail to recognise multiple influences on practice will inevitably founder.

The potential for a clash of values with humanistic approaches in general practice needs to be addressed.[9,10] Research evidence is cited mainly in relation to the prevention, diagnosis, prognosis, treatment and rehabilitation of disease, but this is only one type of knowledge available to health professionals.[11,12] The humanistic approaches focus on the unique personal experience of the patient and the need for the health professional to consider the whole person and the underlying reason for the consultation. The understanding of the life experience ("biography") of the patient is important for the appropriate management of illness – the subjective experience of the individual of being unwell. There is no inherent contradiction between the appropriate use of published research, the use of the patient's life story and the practitioner's emotional and intuitive reaction to it. As "the guardian of the interface between illness and disease",[13] the general practitioner needs to be competent in dealing with both. Indeed, there is some evidence that a patient-centred approach, in which the practitioner explores the patient's experience of illness and the outcomes that they consider to be important, may improve care.[14]

In the scenario shown in Box 12.1, the patient was helped to understand how her symptoms could be linked to her life experiences. The interpretation, although perceived as helpful, was not sufficient to stop her symptoms but enabled her to accept a behavioural intervention for which there is good research evidence of effectiveness.[15] In other cases, interpretation may be sufficient in itself.

Finally, both illness and disease need to be addressed in general practice research. The failure to do so exacerbates the false antithesis between the science and art of medicine. In general practice, "much of the illness that patients bring to professionals is not directly related to disease states that are amenable to biomedical intervention".[16] This observation underscores the need for better information to improve communication between patients and health professionals and also the therapeutic potential of psychological and social interventions. The inclusion of the findings of qualitative research in evidence-based medicine will go some way to addressing legitimate concerns about the limited application of

---

Box 12.1   Case study 1

A 35-year-old woman with two young children presented with a complaint of frequent palpitations for which she had seen another partner in the practice and been referred to a cardiologist who, after appropriate investigation, could find no physical cause for the palpitations. The episodes of palpitations were accompanied by severe anxiety, sweating and light-headedness and the general practitioner thought that she was suffering from panic disorder. In an attempt to elucidate what lay behind her symptoms, the general practitioner asked her about any significant events in her life over the few months since she had been having her symptoms. The patient mentioned that her mother had recently gone back to live abroad, adding "she is my adoptive mother". It transpired that she had been given up for adoption between the ages of 2 and 3 by her "real" mother who had given birth to her at the age of 14. She still had memories of the separation. Despite a period of adolescent conflict, she had become close to her adoptive mother. The practitioner suggested to the patient that her recent separation from her adoptive mother may have rekindled some of the emotions she felt at being separated from her real mother at a young age. The patient was able to make a link between her current symptoms of anxiety and panic and the separations that she had experienced. The practitioner also pointed out how the physical symptoms that she was experiencing were related to her feelings of intense anxiety. The patient appeared reassured but at the follow up consultation 3 weeks later, she reported that she was still having some panic attacks. The practitioner then suggested that she might be helped by cognitive behavioural therapy directed towards the panic disorder and, whilst waiting for this, her symptoms might be improved by taking β-blockers. Eight weeks later, after seeing a clinical psychologist, she reported that the symptoms had greatly improved and she had had no further panic attacks.

---

epidemiological research to the general practice consultation.[17,18]

The use of evidence in the consultation

Some commentators have seen the main constraints to evidence-based general practice as being practical ones.[19] It is not feasible or necessary to apply the full five-step process to all clinical problems although it is clearly important that the logical basis of the approach is understood.[20] The undifferentiated nature of symptoms in general practice and the need to consider illness as well as disease do not imply that general practitioners should be less rigorous than hospital doctors. On the contrary, they need to make use of a wider range of research findings commensurate with the spectrum of problems encountered. A checklist for individual consultations

---

Box 12.2 Is your practice evidence based? A context-specific checklist for individual clinical encounters

Have you:

(1) Identified and prioritised the clinical, psychological, social and other problems, taking into account the patient's perspective?
(2) Performed a sufficiently competent and complete examination to establish the likelihood of competing diagnoses?
(3) Considered additional problems and risk factors?
(4) Where necessary, sought relevant evidence – from systematic reviews, guidelines, clinical trials and other sources?
(5) Assessed and taken into account the completeness, quality and strength of the evidence, and its relevance to this patient?
(6) Presented the pros and cons of the different options to the patient in a way he/she can understand, and incorporated the patient's utilities into the final recommendations?

---

has been suggested for determining whether practice is evidence-based (Box 12.2).[17]

Perhaps the most overwhelming barrier to effective application of evidence in practice is the sheer volume of information being published, amounting to more than two million articles annually.[21] Most general practitioners probably spend considerably less than 2 hours a week reading clinical journals,[19] whereas it has been suggested that a general physician would need to read 19 articles a day 365 days a year to keep up to date.[22] This implies an even greater load for general practitioners. Studies of the information sources of general practitioners have suggested that they tend to rely on colleagues, textbooks and journals.[23] Many of the most frequently read publications are "popular" medical journals which are frequently not peer reviewed. The origin of the information arising from these various sources is largely from research; however, in reaching the general practitioner it has been subject to filtering processes of varying quality.

In order to improve the quality of research based information, the UK NHS Centre for Reviews and Dissemination has published a range of systematic reviews on a number of topics, some of which are highly relevant to primary care[24] and the Cochrane Library has become widely available and is being steadily refined for the use of clinicians.[25]

There are a number of difficulties in accessing appropriate research based information in primary care. Although the quality and presentation is improving, there are still major gaps where no systematic review or well-designed trial exists. This is, in part, due to the underinvestment in primary care research which has resulted in some important conditions being relatively neglected and some studies of common conditions which are generally managed in primary care being undertaken in a hospital setting involving selected populations of patients who may not be representative of those encountered by general practitioners.[26] In part, the dearth of research based information also reflects the great deal of work that remains to be undertaken in reviewing the relevant research literature in a systematic fashion. Identification of trials in general practice may be problematical as they are scattered through the medical literature and not confined to general practice/primary care journals.[27]

Pharmaceutical industry representatives are an important source of information for many general practitioners. A US study by Ziegler et al. (1995) showed that 1 in 10 statements from representatives were in contradiction with the company's own literature and in each case the statements were favourable to the product being marketed.[28] General practitioners need to consider the safety, tolerability, effectiveness and price (STEP) of the treatment being marketed, comparing the new drug where possible to the currently best available treatment. They need to put pharmaceutical representatives to work to ensure that appropriate information is unearthed or acknowledged to be absent.[29]

Without detracting from the real contributions of the pharmaceutical industry to health, it is also clear that a number of problems may arise when sole reliance is placed on studies funded by the pharmaceutical industry in deciding on the value of a particular treatment.[30] In addition, there appears to be an association between single pharmaceutical company sponsorship and a lack of peer review in symposia proceedings and "throwaway" journals.[31] Finally, when those undertaking meta-analyses or systematic reviews attempt to obtain detailed information from pharmaceutical companies it is frequently not forthcoming.[32]

Many general practitioners now use computers in their day-to-day work and most are familiar with MEDLINE. Librarians and medical academics are increasingly providing opportunities to teach general practitioners bibliographic search skills, and some general practitioners now have electronic links from their surgeries, making office-based searching a possibility (see Chapter 3). Free access to MEDLINE is now available through some organisations and professional societies and new sources of relevant information appear regularly on the Internet, including evidence-based guidelines and reports, lists of resources and learning opportunities.

Studies in the USA have shown that teaching critical appraisal skills can improve reading habits, and appreciation of epidemiological concepts.[33-35] Such courses need to encompass not only quantitative research designs, but also qualitative methods. Although a direct link with performance has not been demonstrated, a number of initiatives have been set up to help improve the capacity of general practitioners to determine the validity and applicability of the findings of research. In recognition of the importance of these new skills, the Royal College of General Practitioners in the UK now includes a section on reading papers in their membership examination.[36] However, all too often critical appraisal is used as a way of demonstrating the limitations of papers and does not necessarily assist the practitioner in knowing how to use research evidence.[37]

In the case of general practice, the issues of generalisability and applicability of research findings (external validity) may be as important as internal validity. Generalisability refers to the suitability for implementation in a given setting but without specifying in which circumstances the research evidence is particularly relevant, while applicability relates the research findings to the specific circumstances of the individual patient. Applicability of research is of particular relevance to general practice as, historically, so many studies have taken place in the hospital sector.[38] Although relative risk reduction resulting from a specific intervention in patients from general practice may be similar to that in patients recruited from hospital outpatients, the number needed to treat (NNT) may be greater because of lower absolute risk of an adverse event, as individuals at higher risk are more likely to be referred to hospital.[39] Other patient characteristics such as co-morbidity might also limit the applicability of particular interventions.

It has been suggested that the question we should ask ourselves is "are the patients so different from my patients that I could not apply the study results in my practice?"[40] Using the example of trials of therapeutic interventions, there are a number of components to this question of applicability.

- Is the absolute risk of an adverse event as a result of the underlying disease in this patient likely to be similar to those patients in the study?
- Is the relative risk reduction as a result of treatment likely to be similar?
- Is there any co-morbidity or contraindication which may reduce the benefit?
- Are there any social or cultural factors which might, for example, affect treatment suitability or acceptability?
- What are the patient's and, where relevant, their family's views about the appropriateness of treatment?

It is clear that increasing availability of information and consumerism is shifting the *emphasis* of doctor–patient decision making from more paternalistic transfer of information to one of informed choice.[41] In the case of cardiovascular disease, easy-to-use charts[42] and computer programs[43] have become available to allow rapid calculation of the absolute risk of adverse events in individuals, and of NNTs for groups of patients, so enabling practitioners to give patients more precise information about the risks and benefits of treatment than was possible previously. Also, interactive technologies are being investigated as aids to shared decision making. For example, interactive multimedia programmes on management options for hormone replacement therapy and for benign prostatic hypertrophy have been popular with patients and doctors and have contributed to shared decision making.[44,45] Other investigators are piloting interactive programmes which might be accessed via the Internet. Subject to proper evaluation, such decision aids could provide a cost-effective and practical source of decision support to patients faced with difficult treatment choices in health care.

Much more work is needed to make research evidence directly available to patients. Important initiatives include the provision of information leaflets on pregnancy and childbirth through the Midwives Information and Resource Service Project in the UK,[46] but unfortunately, many sources of information intended for patients omit relevant detail, fail to give a balanced view of the effectiveness of different treatment options and ignore uncertainties.[47]

Influencing the delivery and organisation of care

A difficulty in implementing research based change in practice is the frequent need to influence the organisation and delivery of services as a result of research. This applies even in relatively simple cases such as the prescription of a new drug. The concept of evidence-based medicine emphasises change in practice in response to research findings at the level of the individual consultation of the patient with the health professional. In many incidences, however, the change may have far-reaching implications for a number of members of the primary care team and requires a change in practice policy about how to manage a specific condition. For example, attempts to increase prescription of steroid inhalers in patients with asthma have implications for practice nurses, patients and possibly reception staff, as well as general practitioners. In order to institute change effectively, it may be necessary to alter repeat prescription procedures, improve the quality of information to patients and influence practice nurses who, in the UK system, undertake registration medical checks on patients and, in many instances, run asthma clinics.

In instituting change within practices in response to research based information a number of factors need consideration. These include:

- the nature of the "message"
- which processes in the practice need to be changed
- the key players who can promote or retard change
- the barriers to and levers for change
- the specific interventions which can promote change
- how change can be monitored.

The message and its presentation

In order to make the best use of information to be implemented, a number of steps must be taken, such as clarification of the nature of the message, its scientific basis and to whom it is directed. The content of the message will be determined by evidence of a gap between research findings and clinical practice.

Aspects include:

- scope and content
- scientific (internal) validity
- generalisability and applicability (external validity)
- target audience
- channels for dissemination
- format and presentation
- mechanisms for updating.

In presenting the message, the strength of evidence for specific recommendations should be made explicit. In this way, concerns about "clinical freedom" and professional autonomy may be assuaged. The message is rarely an absolute one and guidelines are to *assist* practitioners in making specific clinical decisions (see Chapter 9). This is because guidelines and other decision support aids can rarely encompass the full range of clinical situations that may confront the practitioner and influence whether or not a given intervention is used in a specific circumstance.

A number of checklists are now available which can help clinicians appraise clinical guidelines. Primary criteria for a good guideline are that the important options and outcomes in the decision process are considered and the evidence on which the guideline is drawn is gathered in an explicit and systematic way. Additional criteria are that the relative values of different outcomes are considered and that the guidelines are regularly updated. Finally, they should be peer reviewed and piloted to ensure that they are relevant and appropriate to the clinical setting and patient group to which they are to be applied.[48,49]

Involving the key players

It is important to involve all the key players at the outset, i.e. those who may implement (or oppose) change. Failure to involve key players may result in rapid demise of an initiative as a result of active or passive opposition. The key players are likely to vary according to the processes that need to be changed, which in turn depend on the chosen topic. In addition to the core members of the primary care team – general practitioners, nurses, reception and administrative staff – they may also include: the local general practitioner tutor if, for example, it is intended to get approval for the postgraduate education allowance for specific practice-based activities; hospital colleagues, if the management of a condition spans the primary/secondary care interface; and psychologists and community psychiatric nurses, for example, if the intention is to make available cognitive behavioural interventions to patients with phobias and other psychological disorders.[15] In the commissioning role of primary care, influence on hospital specialties is particularly important and involving the local health authority at an early stage should ensure that the message given is a consistent one.

Barriers to change

The next step is to identify the barriers to change involving the key players (see also p 109). There are a number of ways of classifying barriers to change. Some examples of potential barriers are given in Box 12.3.

Time constraints, real or perceived, are often of key importance in preventing or retarding the process of change. Many general practitioners have felt under increasing pressure in recent years and this may be partly ascribed to the impact of changes in health policy on primary care, such as the general practitioner contract of 1990 in the UK. Unfortunately, many of these changes were not based on good evidence from research[50,51] and have probably inhibited developments to promote evidence-based practice. Time constraints may be addressed by making better use of time currently spent on continuing education, clinical audit and professional reading as well as ultimately reducing ritualistic activities for which there is no good basis, such as routine urine testing of healthy adults.[52] On occasion, the practitioner may have an adverse early experience with a new intervention, for example, a patient who has a severe gastrointestinal haemorrhage having been put on anticoagulants in order to prevent stroke in atrial fibrillation. Such experiences of a specific intervention can constitute a barrier to change. It is therefore important to examine the overall risks and benefits of a specific intervention and to supplement trial data with data from well-designed observational studies that may more closely approximate to the conditions of day-to-day practice than a randomised trial.[53]

In order to ensure potential barriers are fully identified and steps to overcome them are taken, the key players should agree on the important barriers and how they can be overcome, including the potential levers and specific interventions to promote change.[54]

Levers for change include existing mechanisms that can be used to promote and reinforce the desired change. These might, for example, encompass the use of educational allowances to support programmes aimed at promoting the use of research findings, the inclusion of a section on critical appraisal and the appropriate use of information from research

---

Box 12.3 Examples of potential barriers to change

Practice environment
- Limitations of time
- Practice organisation, for example, lack of disease registers or mechanisms to monitor repeat prescribing

Educational environment
- Inappropriate continuing education and failure to link up with programmes to promote quality of care
- Lack of incentives to participate in effective educational activities

Health care environment
- Lack of financial resources
- Fee for service systems rewarding quantity rather than appropriateness of care
- Lack of defined practice populations
- Health policies which promote ineffective or unproven activities
- Failure to provide practitioners with access to appropriate information

Social environment
- Influence of media in creating demands/beliefs
- Impact of disadvantage on access to care

Practitioner factors
- Obsolete knowledge
- Influence of opinion leaders
- Beliefs and attitudes, for example, related to previous adverse experience of innovation

Patient factors
- Demands for care
- Perceptions/cultural beliefs about appropriate care

Note: Factors that in some circumstances may be perceived as barriers to change can also be levers for change. For example, patients may influence practitioners' behaviour towards clinically effective practice by requesting interventions of proven effectiveness; practitioners may be influenced positively by opinion leaders.

---

in the management of patients in undergraduate and postgraduate examinations. In some countries fee-for-service systems may provide a perverse incentive to undertake inappropriate procedures but can also be used to provide a positive incentive such as the use of target payments to reward attainment of a high level of coverage of selected preventive activities (cervical cytology and immunisation in the UK).

Interventions to change practice

At this stage, if the process continues to be feasible, it is helpful to identify specific interventions which can be used to promote change (see Chapter 8). Different interventions are likely to be suitable according to the problem. For example, where a limited number of tasks need to be repeated at specific time intervals, such as fundoscopy for diabetic patients or measures of diabetic control, a prompting/reminder approach may be best. Computerised templates, available on some general practitioner computer systems, can be used to undertake this task (see Chapter 10). Where complex organisational change is involved the practice team should actively plan, implement and monitor change.

The evidence for the effectiveness of different interventions on professional practice is of variable quality and as much of the work has been undertaken in North America its generalisability to other countries and settings is still unclear (see Chapter 8). Nevertheless it is widely accepted that merely circulating information on a topic is unlikely to change practice appreciably. In the UK, the NHS Research and Development Programme has initiated a portfolio of studies to evaluate different methods of promoting the uptake of research findings.[55] This should substantially improve our knowledge in the foreseeable future.

Guidelines are widely used in attempts to change professional practice and have probably been the most extensively evaluated approach. There is good evidence (see Chapter 9) that they can have substantial impact on practice if they are disseminated using an effective strategy, for example using an active educational intervention. Amongst those approaches to improve the implementation of guidelines that have been investigated (see above), social influence approaches have shown promise in some circumstances. Social influence refers to the process in which "the behaviour of one person has the effect or intention of changing how another person behaves, feels or thinks about something".[56] Social influence approaches acknowledge the importance of shared belief and assumptions, organisational culture and group norms of behaviour. Such processes operate, for example, when a new partner enters a practice or in a group of trainees. Different social influence approaches can be used to promote evidence-based practice according to the setting, i.e. individual small group, larger groups and populations. Some social influence interventions, such as the use of opinion leaders, have not consistently affected behaviour and it seems unlikely that such an approach would work in primary care given the difficulty of identifying and keeping up to date the identification of opinion leaders. A more promising approach is that of "academic detailing", which is the transmission of information from a trained individual (often a pharmacist) to an individual or small group of health professionals. Although this approach particularly emphasises the transmission of information that parallels that used by the pharmaceutical industry, it also incorporates aspects of social influence, for example by emphasising the degree to which other local practitioners are changing their behaviour in the desired direction. It has been effective in reducing inappropriate prescribing and to a lesser extent for increasing preventive activities. [57]

As standard continuing education activities such as lectures, conferences and educational materials appear to have little impact on practice, better use could be made of other approaches such as practice based small-group work which incorporates the use of patient-specific reminders to health professionals where appropriate (see Chapter 11). Dissemination of systematic reviews and evidence-based guidelines could be integrated into the system of continuing medical education for general practitioners. Review in peer learning groups might be the means by which general practitioners become familiar with critical appraisal of summarised information. Combining audit with continuing education has shown mixed results and a number of questions remain about how to enhance effectiveness, including the optimum timing and duration of feedback and the degree to which the involvement of practice teams in designing the

---

Box 12.4 Case study 2

There is extensive evidence that angiotensin-converting enzyme (ACE) inhibitors can improve quality of life and survival and reduce hospital admissions in patients with chronic heart failure and they have been the subject of a systematic review.[59] Nevertheless a minority of patients in primary care have been offered appropriate medication.[60] A practice therefore wishes to improve prescribing for this condition and decides to develop a strategy for existing patients with chronic heart failure along the following lines:

- **Message** – identify patients on loop diuretics. Determine whether they have chronic heart failure by using echocardiography. If no contraindications start on ACE inhibitors observing appropriate precautions to prevent first dose phenomenon. Refer to cardiologist for supervised administration if at high risk of such a reaction using agreed criteria. Monitor renal function.
- **Key players** – general practitioners, receptionists (repeat prescription requests), local cardiologist, echocardiography technician.
- **Barriers** – lack of access to echocardiography. Concerns about initiating ACE inhibitors in primary care.
- **Lever for change** – commissioning of echocardiography open access service.
- **Potential interventions** – guidelines, educational meetings, reminders to general practitioner when filling repeat prescriptions for loop diuretics, feedback to general practitioners on numbers of patients on ACE inhibitors in practice, patient information about change in medication.

The team also wishes to determine how effective the strategy has been in improving practice and therefore repeats the initial audit of those on loop diuretics after 1 year.

---

feedback influences its impact. Primary care teams need to participate actively in the change process if feedback of information from patients is to be an effective means of changing practice. Where practices are actively involved in audit, it seems logical to address gaps in practice by linking education programmes to clinical audit (see Chapter 7). An example of a programme that has made such links is the Australian Quality Assurance and Continuing Education Programme.[58]

Two case studies (Boxes 12.4 and 12.5) may help to illustrate some of the issues involved in promoting implementation of change in primary care. In addition, both of these scenarios illustrate the importance of relationships with secondary care professionals and the importance of access to appropriate diagnostic facilities that may be obtained through the commissioning process, and thus they indicate how commissioning of services may be a lever for change. (In the UK, many general practitioners have been involved in commissioning of hospital services as fundholders with their own practice budget or as part of various commissioning groups. The role and effectiveness of commissioning in promoting evidence-based practice is still open to debate. The second of the two scenarios (Box 12.5)

Box 12.5   Case study 3

A practice nurse attended a short course on the management of diabetes. On her return she requested that, together with one of the general practitioners and the practice manager, she should be made responsible for the organisation of routine care to diabetic patients in the practice. They decided to focus initially on the prevention of visual impairment by regular fundoscopy. The group was aware of guidelines on the topic[61] which had been based on research evidence and adapted these for local use:

- **Message** – all diabetic patients should have an annual fundoscopic examination and be referred to an ophthalmologist if any significant abnormality is detected.
- **Key players** – general practitioners, practice nurses, receptionists, ophthalmologist, optometrist, patients.
- **Barriers** – patients may be unaware of need for eye checks, failure of doctors and receptionists to check whether patient has had annual eye check before giving repeat prescription, general practitioners lack training for fundoscopy, nurse fails to note whether eye examination has been done when performing routine checks, ophthalmologist has long waiting list.
- **Levers** – commission local optometrist to provide fundoscopy service after appropriate training. Practice remunerated to provide structured diabetes care.
- **Potential interventions** – information for patients; prompting system for general practitioners, using practice computer to develop template for diabetic care; colour code diabetic patients' records to remind receptionist; recall by nurses of all patients not seen within 1 year; team meetings to agree on guidelines and monitor progress.

also illustrates the potential importance of non-medical members of the team as change agents.

Conclusions

The pace of development of medical knowledge poses a considerable challenge to primary care, significantly greater even than that to hospital practice because of the wider range of conditions seen by general practitioners and the relative dearth of primary care research. More resources will need to be devoted to research on the diagnosis, prognosis, prevention and treatment of disease in primary care and on systematically reviewing what has already been done.

In addition to the many other contributions that it can make to the understanding of health and health care, qualitative research can illuminate the doctor–patient relationship by improving understanding of how patients' life experiences and health beliefs influence their presenting complaint and the treatment which they consider is appropriate for their condition, thus opening the way for better informed decisions in the consultation and improved resolution of the patients' problems. It can also give information about the attitudes of health professionals to the use of research evidence[59] and has an important role in improving the prospects for more effective practice.[17]

In order to use research evidence more effectively in practice, primary care teams need valid and relevant information synthesised in a user-friendly format. This is beginning to become available through the Cochrane Collaboration and other sources but many practitioners do not have adequate support from library services for document retrieval and assistance with searches. Information providers are likely to be increasingly seen as members of the extended primary care team.

Despite considerable investment in information technology and evidence that decision support, even of simple kinds such as prompting and reminder systems, can promote more effective practice, we still lack adequate systems. However, the situation is changing rapidly and will undoubtedly improve in the foreseeable future.

It has been suggested that the process by which innovations are taken up within social systems is a stepwise process which includes: the acquisition of knowledge, persuasion of the practitioner that the innovation is appropriate for use, the decision to use it, the act of implementation and finally confirmation that the innovation has become an accepted part of practice.[62] Better understanding of the factors which promote and retard organisational change in primary care teams should be given higher priority.

Although much of the work on factors that promote or inhibit the uptake of innovations has been undertaken in other sectors, some of the implications may be relevant to general practice. This work is an important reminder that social and organisational factors may be important determinants of change, in addition to the characteristics of the innovation itself, such as its complexity (whether the practitioner feels it is straightforward to implement), trialability (whether the practitioner can try out the innovation before adopting it for routine practice) and observability (whether the practitioner can observe the results of the innovation on the patients of other doctors). There is some evidence that these factors may be relevant in the health sector with regard to adherence to practice guidelines.[63]

The growth of accessible sources of information for patients based on research evidence has the potential to influence the doctor–patient relationship profoundly. General practitioners are likely to find themselves increasingly acting as information brokers – helping patients critically appraise information they receive about their condition from the media and their social networks and pointing them to sources of high-quality information which meet their needs. There are also opportunities for new partnerships with user groups, many of which have a growing interest in drawing together rigorous information about effective practice in their area of interest. In the UK, for example, the Health Information Quality Centre has been funded by the Department of Health to help patients make informed decisions and will act as a resource for patients, user groups and health professionals alike.[64]

A change in professional culture invariably takes time, but by offering practitioners the skills to respond creatively to changes in knowledge and to integrate research findings into their day-to-day practice, the concepts of evidence-based practice should help to counter the decay in the applicability of knowledge gained during undergraduate and postgraduate training, improve the quality of services offered and maximise the health gains to our patients.

References

1 Leach E. *Social anthropology.* Glasgow: Fontana, 1982: pp 38–9.
2 Sackett DL, Haynes RB, Guyatt GH, Tugwell P. *Clinical epidemiology: a basic science for clinical medicine.* Boston: Little, Brown, 1991.
3 Toon P. *What is good general practice?* Occasional paper No 65. London: Royal College of General Practitioners, 1994.
4 Balint M. *The doctor, his patient and the illness.* London: Pitman Medical, 1957.
5 Stewart M, Brown JB, Western WW, McWhitney IR, McWilliam CL, Freeman TR. *Patient-centred medicine – transforming the clinical method.* California: Sage, 1995.
6 Hart JT. *A new kind of doctor.* London: Merlin Press, 1988.
7 Gillam S, Plamping D, McClenahan J, Harries J, Epstein L. *Community-oriented primary care.* London: King's Fund, 1994.
8 Helman C. *Culture, health and illness.* Oxford: Butterworth-Heinemann, 1994.
9 Charlton R. Balancing science and art in primary care research: past and

present. *Br J Gen Pract* 1995;45:639-40.
10 Smith BH, Taylor RJ. Medicine – a healing or a dying art? *Br J Gen Pract* 1996;46:249-51.
11 Naylor CD. Grey zones of clinical medicine: some limits to evidence-based medicine. *Lancet* 1996;345:840-2.
12 Sullivan FM, MacNaughton RJ. Evidence in consultations: interpreted and individualised. *Lancet* 1996;348:941-3.
13 Heath I. The future of general practice. In Lock S, ed. *Eighty-five not out.* London: King's Fund, 1993, pp 19-22.
14 Stewart M, Brown JB, Weston WW, McWhinney JR. *Studies of health outcomes and patient-centred communication. Patient-centred medicine.* California: Sage, 1995.
15 Mattick RP, Andrews G, Hadzi-Pavlovic D, Christensen H. Treatment of panic and agoraphobia: an integrative review. *J Nerv Ment Dis* 1991;78:567-76.
16 Pratt J. *Practitioners and practices – a conflict of values?* Oxford: Radcliffe Medical Press, 1995.
17 Greenhalgh T. Is my practice evidence-based? *BMJ* 1996;313:957-8.
18 Risdale L. Evidence-based learning for general practice. *Br J Gen Pract* 1996;46:503.
19 Dawes MG. On the need for evidence-based general and family practice. *Evidence-Based Med* 1996;1:68-9.
20 Felton A, Lister G. *Consider the evidence.* Uxbridge: Coopers & Lybrand, 1996.
21 Mulrow CD. Rationale for systematic reviews. *BMJ* 1994;309:597-9.
22 Davidoff F, Haynes RB, Sackett DL, Smith R. Evidence-based medicine. A new journal to help doctors identify the information they need (editorial). *BMJ* 1995;310:1085-6.
23 Urquhart C, Hepworth JB. *The value to clinical decision making of information supplied by NHS Library and information services.* British library R & D report 6205. London: The British Library Board, 1995.
24 NHS Centre for Reviews and Dissemination. University of York. www.york.uc.uk/inst/crd/ehcb.htm.
25 *Cochrane Library.* Update Software. Oxford, 2000.
26 Sweeney KG, Gray DJP, Steele RJF, Evans PH. Caution needed in introducing warfarin treatment (commentary). *BMJ* 1995;311:560-1.
27 Silagy C. Developing a register of randomised controlled trials in primary care. *BMJ* 1993;306:879-900.
28 Ziegler MG, Lew P, Singer BC. The accuracy of drug information from pharmaceutical sales representatives. *JAMA* 1995;273:1296-8.
29 Shaughnessy AF, Slawson DC. Pharmaceutical representatives: Effective if used with caution. *BMJ* 1996;312:1494.
30 Bero LA, Rennie D. Influences on the quality of published drug studies. *Int J Tech Assess Health Care* 1996;12:209-37.
31 Rennie D, Bero LA. Throw it away Sam: the controlled circulation journals. *Council Biological Editors'Views* 1990;13:31-5.
32 Freemantle N, Haines A, Mason J, Eccles M. CONSORT – An important step towards evidence-based health care. *Ann Intern Med* 1997;126:81-2.
33 Linzer M, Brown JT, Frazier LM, DeLong ER, Siegel WC. Impact of a medical journal club on house-staff reading habits, knowledge and critical appraisal skills. *JAMA* 1988;260:2537-41.
34 Bennett KJ, Sackett DL, Haynes RB, Neufeld VR, Tugwell P, Roberts R. A controlled study of teaching critical appraisal to medical students. *JAMA* 1987;257:2451-545.
35 Seelig CB. Affecting residents' literature-reading attitudes, behaviours, and

knowledge through journal club intervention. *J Gen Intern Med* 1991;6:330–4.
36 Lockie C, ed. *Examination for membership of the Royal College of General Practitioners (MRCGP)*. London: RCGP, 1990.
37 Hyde CJ. Using the evidence. A need for quantity not quality? *Int J Tech Assess Health Care* 1995;12:280–7.
38 Wilson S, Delaney B, Roalfe A, *et al*. Randomised controlled trials in primary care: case study. *BMJ* 2000;321:24–7.
39 Smeeth L, Haines A, Ebrahim S. Numbers needed to treat derived from meta-analyses – sometimes informative, usually misleading. *BMJ* 1999;318:1548–51.
40 Evidence-based Medicine Working Group. Evidence-based medicine. A new approach to teaching the practice of medicine. *JAMA* 1992;268:2420–5.
41 O'Connor AM. Consumer-patient decision support in the new millennium: where should our research take us? *Can J Nurs Res* 1997;29:7–12.
42 Jackson R, Barham P, Bills J, *et al*. Management of raised blood pressure in New Zealand: a discussion document. *BMJ* 1993;307:107–10.
43 Hingorani AD, Vallance P. A simple computer programme for guiding management of cardiovascular risk factors and prescribing. *BMJ* 1999;318:101–5.
44 Murray E, Davis H, See Tai S, Gray A, Coulter A, Haines A. A randomised controlled trial of an interactive multimedia decision aid on hormone replacement therapy in primary care. Accepted for publication. www.bmj.com.
45 Murray E, Davis H, See Tai S, Coulter A, Gray A, Haines A. A randomised controlled trial of an interactive multimedia decision aid on benign prostatic hypertrophy in primary care. Accepted for publication. www.bmj.com.
46 Midwives Information and Resource Service. *Informed choice*. Bristol: 1995.
47 Coulter A, Entwhistle V, Gilbert D. *Informing patients. An assessment of the quality of patient information materials*. London: King's Fund, 1998.
48 Hayward RSA, Wilson MC, Tunis SR, Bass EB, Guyatt G. Users' guides to the medical literature. VII. How to use clinical practice guidelines. Are the recommendations valid? *JAMA* 1995;274:570–4.
49 Wilson MC, Hayward RSA, Tunis SR, Bass EB, Guyatt G. Users' guides to the medical literature. VIII. What are the recommendations and will they help you in caring for your patients? *JAMA* 1995;274:1630–2.
50 Morrell DC. Role of research in development of organisation and structure of general practice. *BMJ* 1991;302:1313–16.
51 Perkins E. Screening elderly people: a review of the literature in the light of the new general practitioner contract. *Br J Gen Pract* 1991;41:382–5.
52 Fowler G, Mant D. Urine analysis for glucose and protein: are the requirements of the new contract sensible? *BMJ* 1990;300:1053–5.
53 Palareti G, Leali N, Coccheri S, Poggi M, Marotti C. Bleeding complications of oral anticoagulant treatment: an inception – cohort, prospective collaborative study (ISCOAT). *Lancet* 1996;348:423–8.
54 Baker R, Sorrie R, Reddish S, Hearnshaw H, Roberston N. The facilitation of multiprofessional clinical audit in primary health care teams – from audit to quality assurance. *J Interprofessional Care* 1995;9:237–44.
55 Report of Advisory Group to the Central Research and Development Committee. *Methods to promote the implementation of research findings in the NHS – priorities for evaluation*. Leeds: Department of Health, 1995.
56 Mittman BS, Tonesk X, Jacobson PD. Implementing clinical practice guidelines: social influence strategies and practitioner behaviour change. *Qual Rev Bull* 1992;18:413–21.
57 Bero L, Freemantle N, Grilli R, *et al*. Closing the gap between research and practice: an overview of the systematic reviews of the interventions to promote

implementation of research findings by health care professionals. In: Haines A, Donald A, eds. *Getting research findings into practice*. London: BMJ Books, 1998.

58 Salisbury C. The Australian Quality Assurance and Continuing Education Programme as a model for reaccreditation of general practitioners in the United Kingdom. *Br J Gen Pract* 1997;47:319–22.

59 Garg G, Yusuf S. Overview of randomised controlled trials of ACE inhibitors on mortality and morbidity in patients with heart failure. *JAMA* 1995;273:1450–6.

60 Mair FS, Crowley TS, Bundred PE. Prevalence, aetiology and management of heart failure in general practice. *Br J Gen Pract* 1996;46:77–9.

61 Scottish Intercollegiate Guidelines Network. *The care of diabetic patients in Scotland. Prevention of visual impairment*. SIGN publication no 4. Edinburgh: Royal College of Physicians, 1996.

62 Rogers EM. *Diffusion of innovations*. New York: Free Press, 1983.

63 Grilli R, Lomas J. Evaluating the message: the relationship between compliance rate and the subject of a practice guideline. *Med Care* 1994;132:202–13.

64 Stocking B. Partners in care. *Health Management* 1997;1:12–13.

Appendix 1: Using MEDLINE to search for evidence (Ovid software) – some background information and sample searches

BARBARA CUMBERS AND REINHARD WENTZ

Note: The information in this appendix is still valid in 2001 and helpful to those who conduct exhaustive, systematic searches and wish to understand the search process in detail. However, evidence-based health care (EBHC) searching is moving away from complex searches on large medical databases with their poor signal-to-noise ratio to extracting, synthesising, evaluating databases such as COCHRANE, DARE and TRIP (see Appendix 2). Here the use of one or two distinct words, selected from the clinical scenario, usually generates small sets of hits, which are often arranged by their level of evidence.

If you find the search process as outlined below too complicated you may also want to try the "Clinical Queries" question on PubMed (the full MEDLINE version, freely available on the Internet – see Appendix 2 for URL and detailed description). Here "filter terms" for a therapeutic, diagnostic, risk, or prognostic clinical scenario are added "automatically". Searches can be entered using natural language/textword terms and can then be adjusted for sensitivity and specificity.

The material in this Appendix is based on the Windows version of the OVID (CD-Plus) software, version 3.00, and should be easily convertible to other versions of Ovid. The general principles are applicable to other MEDLINE search programs, with modifications. You are advised to consult your local medical librarian.

The MEDLINE database

MEDLINE is compiled by the National Library of Medicine of the USA, and indexes over 3400 journals published in 70 countries. The database is available in three main formats:

- printed (called *Index Medicus*)
- on-line (the whole database from 1966 to date on an Internet server, accessed via the Internet, for example, PubMed, the freely available version of MEDLINE – see Appendix 2)
- CD Rom (the whole database on between 13 and 20 CDs, depending on vendor; Ovid uses 13).

Articles are indexed by a restricted thesaurus of medical terms: MeSH (Medical Subject Headings). The indexers allocate terms from MeSH to each article, often refining them with subheadings (also selected from a restricted list).

MeSH is arranged hierarchically: some terms are more specific subdivisions of others. It is possible to "explode" a term which has more specific terms, so as to include them all. For example, the search statement "explode heart diseases" will find everything indexed under any heart disease term.

The indexers mark some terms (or term subheading combinations) with a * in the record (called "focus" on Ovid). This means that the term is of particular relevance to that article.

In the computer formats (though not on all internet versions), the records are searchable by:

- MeSH terms (the Ovid default search), with or without subheadings
- any words appearing in the record, including authors' names.

The following points should be borne in mind when searching MEDLINE:

- the indexers are fallible, and the indexing is subject to quirks. Thus, not all articles mentioning "heart attack" will be indexed under the equivalent MeSH term (myocardial infarction). To be comprehensive, a search should make use of textwords (words appearing in the title or abstract of the record) as well as terms
- the indexing is specific. An article on endocarditis will be indexed under "endocarditis" or "endocarditis, bacterial", not under "heart diseases" (though "explode heart diseases" would find everything indexed under "endocarditis" – as well as 30 000 other references which you may or may not want!)
- to retrieve meaningful results, searchers must construct search strategies that accurately specify their needs (although they must be

prepared to modify them in the light of interim results)
- although MEDLINE is big (over 8 million records), it is not comprehensive, and many journals are not indexed in it. A comprehensive search should perhaps also include a search of other biomedical databases (see Appendix 2).

How to construct a simple search strategy

Identify the most important concept(s) of your subject

Break your subject down into its component parts, so that it can be entered in a way the computer will understand. The computer understands:

- words or phrases that it can "map" to a MeSH term
- phrases that form a MeSH term (with or without a subheading)
- coded field names (see the full record on page 185–6 for examples of field names)
- link words AND, OR, NOT, and ADJ.

If your subject contains at least two distinct concepts:

- enter each concept separately. Ovid will automatically "map" what you enter to the appropriate MeSH term or will give you a list to choose from
- use the "explode" option if available for each MeSH term
- do not use the "focus" option at this stage
- do not use subheadings at this stage
- combine the concepts (usually with the Boolean operator "AND" which will find those references common to both sets).

You will be astonished how frequently this simple method creates a manageable set of possibly relevant papers. Scan the list of references and "mark" directly relevant ones. Do not routinely rely on the search software to reduce a list of, say, less than 30 papers, to the five papers you expected: use your own judgment.

If you find **more** papers than you expected, or can cope with:

- add another concept and combine concepts with "AND"
- use the "restrict to focus" option for one or more initial MeSH terms
- apply a subheading, or set of subheadings, to one or more terms
- use the "limit" command, for example to age group
- use methodological filters (see pages 180–2).

If you find **fewer** papers than you expected:

- identify a more general MeSH term and explode it
- find related MeSH terms and "or" them together
- combine a MeSH term search with a textword search for each concept, then combine the sets with "or". For textword searching, remember to include spelling variations and the truncation mark ($ in Ovid)
- eliminate less important concepts from your search strategy
- include synonyms
- ensure brackets are used correctly.

If your subject contains only one concept:

- identify its MeSH term. Ovid will "map" it automatically or will ask you to try a synonym
- use suitable subheading(s) when prompted.

If the MeSH term and subheading(s) are selected carefully, this procedure will often create a manageable set of references which you can start scanning for relevant material.

If you find **more** papers than you expected or can cope with:

- add another concept
- use the "restrict to focus" option for the initial MeSH term
- use the "limit" command, for example to age group
- use methodological filters (see pages 180–2).

If your subject contains only one concept which does not yield a suitable MeSH term:

- try a textword search, restricted to the title field (Add ".ti." to the words.)
- check the MeSH terms used by the indexers for any papers found. (If these are not displayed, on the CD Rom version, use the "Options" pull down menu at the top of the screen to add the MeSH terms to the fields displayed; on the on-line version, click on the "Complete Reference" button.)
- search some of the MeSH terms found and build a search strategy using them.

To be as comprehensive as possible:

- always use both MeSH terms and textwords in your search strategy
- look at any related MeSH terms that Ovid suggests in the MeSH "Scope note".

Evidence-based medicine and MEDLINE searches

The concept of evidence-based medicine (or evidence-based health care) advocates that clinical and health care decisions should be based on the best evidence available from critically appraised studies which can be applied to clinical and health care planning questions.

Applied to information retrieval, this concept suggests that a search should concentrate on scientifically valid and relevant literature with direct implications for clinical practice or health care planning.

It would also imply that more use should be made of computerised sources of information which help in the systematic location of relevant information, and in reducing the time lag before, for example, therapies of proven effectiveness are implemented in medical practice.

The MEDLINE indexers now take the concepts of evidence-based health care into account, and a range of subject terms is now available to aid searching for valid and comprehensive studies. Coupled with a highly sensitive subject search, they can be used to find valid and relevant studies.

The following search strategies have been adapted from the "methodologic filters" developed at McMaster University for the greatest sensitivity compatible with specificity and precision. Our adaptations have been made with the aim of reducing the time they take to run. They should be sensitive and specific enough to retrieve substantial studies (on MEDLINE) for many subjects. (The original McMaster filters are available pre-loaded on PubMed under the "Clinical Queries" option.)

The filters should be used in parallel with a subject search which is as sensitive (comprehensive) as possible (see the examples on pages 183–8). It is suggested that you enter the filters on your computer and save them permanently (your librarian may already have done this). You can call them up (from the "File" menu) and run them as appropriate. The sample searches show how they can be used.

These filters are still being developed and may have to be altered or amended if applied to specific clinical questions. They are not definitive or authoritative and their reliability cannot easily be tested.

- Highly sensitive filters can take a long time to run, and have the additional drawback of tending to have a low specificity and precision.
- In adapting the following filters, we have tried to balance time against effectiveness. Our filters are not exhaustive but will (we hope) be practical to use and sensitive enough for most subjects.
- Three versions of some filters are given, to be used as time and subject demand.
- Please consult a medical librarian if you need further advice.

Therapeutic interventions/randomised controlled trials. (What works?)

a A practical, fairly sensitive strategy

1 controlled clinical trials/
2 randomised controlled trials/
3 exp research design/
    (would include "double-blind method", "meta-analysis" and "random allocation" as MeSH terms)
4 multi-center studies/
5 single-blind method/
    (lines 1 to 5 are MeSH terms, including all subheadings)
6 clinical trial.pt.
    (line 6 searches for "clinical trial" as a publication type: it would include "randomised controlled trial" as a publication type)
7 ((single or double or treble or triple) adj5 (mask$ or blind$)).tw.
    (line 7 searches for textwords: a word in the first group must be within 5 words of a word in the second group; $ is the truncation symbol)
8 placebos/ or placebo$.tw.
    (the first is a MeSH term; the second is a textword)
9 or/1-8

b A highly specific strategy

1 exp research design/
2 randomised controlled trial.pt.
3 1 or 2

c A quick one-line strategy

1 clinical trial.pt.

Aetiology. (What causes it? What are the risk factors?)

a A practical, fairly sensitive strategy

1 exp causality/
    (would include "risk factors" and "precipitating factors" as MeSH terms)
2 exp cohort studies/
    (would include "prospective studies" as a MeSH term)
3 exp risk/
    (would include "risk assessment as a MeSH term)
4 exp case-control studies/
    (would include "retrospective studies" as a MeSH term)
5 or/1–4

b A highly specific strategy

1 case-control studies/
2 cohort studies/
3 1 or 2

c A quick one-line strategy

1 risk.tw,hw.

> (would include "risk" in the title or abstract, or as a word in a MeSH term)

Diagnostic procedures

a A practical, fairly sensitive strategy

1 exp "sensitivity and specificity"/

> (*The quotation marks are essential, since the MeSH term contains a Boolean word - "and".*)
>
> (would include "predictive value of tests" as a MeSH term)

2 exp diagnostic errors/

> (would include "false negative reactions" and "observer variation" as MeSH terms)

3 exp mass screening/

> (would include "neonatal screening" and "genetic screening" as MeSH terms)

4 or/1-3

b A highly specific strategy

1 exp "sensitivity and specificity"/

2 (predictive adj5 value$).tw.

3 1 or 2

c A quick one-line strategy

1 sensitivity.tw,hw.

Prognosis

a A practical, fairly sensitive strategy

1 survival rate/

2 disease progression/

3 exp survival analysis/

> (would include "disease-free survival" as a MeSH term)

4 exp cohort studies/

> (would include "longitudinal studies", "follow-up studies" and "prospective studies")

5 exp prognosis/

> (would include "treatment outcome")

6 prognos$.tw.

> (would search for "prognosis" or "prognostic" as words in the title or abstract)

7 or/1-6

b A highly specific strategy

1 exp prognosis/

2 exp survival analysis/
3 1 or 2

c A quick one-line strategy
1 exp cohort studies/

Epidemiology

1 sn.xs.
> (this cryptic line means "find any MeSH term which has a statistical (sn) subheading attached to it (.xs.)"; the statistical subheadings are "statistics" "epidemiology" "ethnology" and "mortality")

Finally two different types of filter, which can be used on any subject search:
> *(These are fairly sensitive strategies, and will run in an acceptable time on most computers: they are not exhaustive.)*

How to find systematic reviews on MEDLINE

1 review, academic.pt.
2 review, tutorial.pt.
3 meta-analysis.pt.
> (lines 1, 2 and 3 search for publication types)
4 (systematic$ adj5 review$).tw.
5 (systematic$ adj5 overview$).tw.
> (lines 4 and 5 search for "systematic" or "systematical" adjacent to "review(s)" or "overview(s)" in the title or the abstract)
6 meta-analysis/
> "meta-analysis" as a MeSH term)
7 meta-analysis.tw.
> "meta-analysis" as a word in the title or the abstract)
8 or/1–7

How to find guidelines and recommendations on MEDLINE

1 guideline.pt.
2 practice guideline.pt.
> lines 1 and 2 search for publication types)
3 (guideline$ or recommend$ or consensus).tw.
4 (standards or parameter$).tw.
> lines 3 and 4 search for words in the title or abstract)
5 exp guidelines/
> searches for "guidelines" or"practice guidelines" as MeSH terms)
6 health planning guidelines/
7 or/1–6

Some examples of MEDLINE searches using filters

The first example is adapted from one given in David Sackett's book *Evidence-based medicine: how to practise and teach EBM* which describes the whole process from presentation to implementation, with comments on methods and results. The book is highly recommended to anyone interested in EBM.

These sample searches aim to show you the thought processes that you should find helpful in searching MEDLINE. Search 1 is explained in detail; searches 2 and 3 more briefly.

Sample search 1: In a patient with mild renal impairment, is there a form of contrast media for intravenous pyelography that lowers the risk of worsening the renal function?

Search strategy: We need information that is about both renal impairment and intravenous pyelography or contrast media, not about each of these individually.

The first step is to select terms from the thesaurus (MeSH). Typing in "renal impairment" leads to a list (from Ovid's mapping process) headed by *kidney diseases; kidney failure, chronic;* and *kidney failure*. A scope note suggests we also try terms listed under *NEPHR-* and *RENAL*. *Kidney diseases* is very general and "exploding" it (see page 176) would include subjects irrelevant to this search. *Kidney failure, chronic* seems too specific and would be included by "exploding" *kidney failure*. The last option seems the best bet, so:

1 exp kidney failure   **10134**

("Exp" at the beginning of a search statement indicates that a MeSH term has been "exploded"; "/" at the end of a search statement indicates that Ovid has searched for a MeSH term with any subheading. You do not have to remember to add these symbols yourself as the mapping and term selection procedure will do it automatically.)

As a result of the suggestion in the scope note, we should look at *nephrology* and *renal* in the Permuted MeSH (from the "Tools" menu at the top of the Ovid search screen). We find that all relevant terms are cross-referenced back to *kidney failure* or one of its specifics, and so have already been included.

We could leave it there and proceed with the next concept, "intravenous pyelography", but we want to be as sensitive as possible, so we need to think of all possible relevant terms and textwords for "renal impairment" that might not have been included so far. Check any synonyms or related terms in the thesaurus and OR any that you find into the search strategy. If you do not find the synonyms in the thesaurus, add them anyway as textwords. Textwords are particularly important for new concepts that indexers have not yet incorporated.

A probably relevant term is "azotaemia". The British spelling maps to **kidney failure, acute** which we have already included, but strangely enough, the American spelling "azotemia" maps to **uremia** which is relevant but which would have been otherwise excluded. As there was a problem with "azotaemia", textwords might be a good idea anyway.

2 exp uremia	1790
3 (azotemi\$ or azotaemi\$).tw	312

Notice that we have not searched for the term **kidney**. This is because indexers use the most specific term available, and if we searched for **contrast agents** and **kidney**, we would probably miss articles on contrast agents in chronic renal failure. If you are not sure which specific term might be best (a problem that indexers have too), select a "parent" term and "explode", as we did with **kidney failure**.

We now follow much the same procedure for "intravenous pyelography", which Ovid maps to urography, but to be thorough we will also include "pyelography" as a textword, truncated (\$) to include various endings and forms:

4 urography/	815
5 pyelogra\$.tw	346

"Contrast media" leads straightforwardly to **contrast media** with a very long list of specifics, making textwords a time-consuming and probably unproductive exercise. More effective to just "explode" it:

6 exp contrast media/	6159

We can now link everything together:

7 (1 or 2 or 3) and (4 or 5 or 6)	141

This interprets as: (all renal failure terms linked by OR) AND (all the contrast media and urography terms linked by OR). OR includes all references in any of the sets, that is, it broadens searches; AND in a search strategy collects only those articles that have both or all terms, so narrowing the search. The brackets tell the computer which operations to perform first.

It would be time-consuming to go through 141 references, so now we need to add our filter(s). Our example is a question of "cause" (does IVP cause, or worsen, renal failure?), so we could run the "Aetiology" filter. It is also a question that lends itself to randomised controlled trials, so we could run the "RCT" ("Therapy") filter too.

That might take too long, so we could try looking for systematic reviews first, by running the "Systematic reviews" filter:

8 review, academic.pt..18859
9 meta-analysis.pt..1670
10 meta-analysis/..1002
11 (systematic$ adj25 review$).tw..609
12 (systematic$ adj25 overview$).tw..79
13 or/8-12 21797

Then AND the result to the earlier result, set 7:

14 13 and 7..12

The search yielded a number of reviews, one of which was a meta-analysis by Barrett and Carlisle (see below). This systematic review indicated that use of low-osmolality contrast media (LOCM) poses a significantly lower risk for worsening renal function, particularly for patients with initial renal impairment.

It is a matter of practice and experience (not to mention luck) in judging whether a "subject" filter is more appropriate than the "Systematic reviews" one. Had we run the "Aetiology" and "RCT" filters on this search, the result would have been 54 references, including the Barrett and Carlisle one. Of course, 54 references would still take time to look through, and you might have decided to run "systematic reviews" against the 54 anyway. The result then would have been five references. including the Barrett and Carlisle one.

The full record of the Barrett and Carlisle reference, as it appears on Ovid MEDLINE, is shown below (the field names are in bold print).

Note the following points:

- some MeSH terms have a * in front of them. These are the terms that the indexers considered most important, and are what Ovid looks for when you ask it to "restrict to focus". The allocation of * status to a term can seem arbitrary in some instances
- The "publication type" field (third from the end) is the field searched by adding ".pt." to a search statement. This field can only be searched in this way; it is not searched by a textword search.

Unique identifier 93288868
Authors Barrett BJ. Carlisle Ej.
Institution Division of Nephrology, Health Sciences Center, St John's, Newfoundland, Canada.
Title Meta-analysis of the relative nephrotoxicity of high- and low-osmolality iodinated contrast media.
Source Radiology. 188(1):171-8, 1993 Jul.
Abbreviated source Radiology. 188(1):171-8, 1993 Jul.
NLM journal code qsh
Journal subset A, C

Country of publication United States
MeSH subject headings Comparative Study; *Contrast Media/ae [Adverse Effects]; Human; Iodine/ae [Adverse Effects]; Iodine/du [Diagnostic Use]; *Kidney Failure/ci [Chemically Induced]; Osmolar Concentration; Support, Non-U.S. Gov't

Abstract To determine whether low-osmolality contrast media (LOCM) are less nephrotoxic than high-osmolality contrast media (HOCM), the authors searched MEDLINE and EMBASE databases and other sources to find randomized trials with data collected on changes in glomerular filtration rate or serum creatinine (SCr) level with LOCM and HOCM. Forty-five trials were found. Data were unavailable from 14 trials. When the P values from the other 31 trials were pooled, an overall P value of 0.02 was found. Among 24 trials with available data, the mean change in SCr was 0.2-6.2 micromol/L less with LOCM than HOCM. Among 25 trials with available data, the pooled odds of a rise in SCr level of more than 44 micromol/L with LOCM was 0.61 (95% confidence interval [CI], 0.48–0.77) times that after HOCM. For patients with existing renal failure, this odds ratio was 0.5 (CI, 0.36–0.68), while it was 0.75 (CI, 0.52–1.1) in patients without prior renal failure. Greater changes in SCr level occurred only in those with existing renal failure and were less common with LOCM (odds ratio, 0.44; CI, 0.26–0.73). Use of LOCM may be beneficial in patients with existing renal failure.

Registry numbers 0 (Contrast Media). 7553-56-2 (Iodine). ISSN 0033-8419
Publication type Journal article. Meta-analysis. Language English.
Entry month 9309.

Sample search 2: Does breastfeeding reduce the risk of breast cancer?

In this sample search, we have not used textwords or looked for synonyms. This is to illustrate how simply and quickly an adequate search can be done when the concepts "map" easily to MeSH terms.

Identify the two important subjects ("breast cancer" and "breastfeeding"), and map them separately: "breast cancer" to:

    1 exp breast neoplasms/ **19112**

and "breastfeeding" conveniently to:

    2 breast feeding/ **2417**

To keep the results as sensitive as possible:
- do **not** focus either MeSH term
- do **not** use subheadings.

    3 1 and 2 ....**32**

Apply the "risk" ("Aetiology") filter:

    4 exp causality/ 22193
    5 exp cohort studies/ 39370
    6 exp, risk/...26212
    7 or/4-6..60367

Then AND that result to the subject search (set 3) (a Boolean AND retrieves the overlap between two sets or two groups):

    8 3 and 7 15

These 15 references contained some substantial studies which were of interest.

Sample search 3: Does MMR cause Crohn's disease?

Test "mmr" and you will find that it maps to a range of MeSH terms, including "measles vaccine", "mumps vaccine ", and "rubella vaccine" – there is no direct MeSH term for it. So try "mmr" in the title field and inspect the MeSH field to confirm that "mmr" is consistently indexed under all three "vaccine" terms:

    1 mmr. ti 36

Looking at some of these references will confirm that those on the combination vaccine of interest are all indexed under all three disease terms and/or the vaccine terms.

    2 measles vaccine and mumps vaccine and rubella
    vaccine/...236
Use set 1 as a control:

    3 1 not 2 4

and you will find that there are still four references which set 2 did not retrieve. Looking at them shows that two are false positives but the other two are relevant.

Amend your search strategy accordingly, i.e. "or" terms in set 2 together, also create a set with the corresponding disease terms (set 5):

    4 measles vaccine/ or mumps vaccine/ or rubella
    vaccine/...838
    5 measles/ or mumps/ or rubella/.......................................1370
    6 4 or 5 1723

Set 6 is a sensitive set of (?nearly) everything potentially relevant to "mmr".

Now combine that set with "Crohn's disease" which maps to:

> **7 Crohn disease/** **2287**
>
> **8 6 and 7** **11**

Set 8 contains 11 references, all of which should be relevant. Should you want more than 11 references (before you include the causality concept), you could try to improve recall by broadening one or more terms (Ovid prompts you to look at broader terms).

Broader terms for "Crohn's disease" are:

> **9 exp inflammatory bowel diseases/** **4327**
>
> **10 exp intestinal diseases/** **39884**

Combined with set 6 ("everything possibly relevant to mmr"), it gives you a wider set of potentially relevant papers (and which by definition includes set 8):

> **11 6 and (9 or 10)** **49**

Now run an "Aetiology" filter:

> **12 exp causality/** **22193**
>
> **13 exp cohort studies/** **39370**
>
> **14 exp risk/** **26212**
>
> **15 or/12-14** **60367**

Then AND the result to the result of the subject search (set 11):

> **16 11 and 15** **15**

and include all of set 8 in your final set:

> **17 16 or 8** **19**

Set 17 should constitute a good list for looking through in MEDLINE and "marking" the highly relevant ones for printing out.

Systematic reviews

Systematic reviews are particularly important in evidence-based care because:

- they help decision makers cope with the sheer volume of published literature by summarising it in a rigorous way
- they adopt a comprehensive strategy for searching for primary studies, including both published and unpublished sources, and explain the criteria for the inclusion or exclusion of any study
- they give a clear, statistical synthesis of the data from eligible studies, and include a structured report of the review.

The filter on page 182 will enable you to find systematic reviews on

MEDLINE. Some other sources of systematic reviews are listed in Appendix 2.

Further reading

Haynes, RB, Wilczyriski NL, McKibbon KA, Walker CJ, Sinclair JC. Developing optimal search strategies for detecting clinically sound studies in MEDLINE. *J Am Med Informatics Assoc* 1994; 1: 447-58.

Sackett DL, Richardson WS, Rosenberg W, Haynes RB. *Evidence-based medicine: how to practice and teach EBM*. London: Churchill Livingstone, 1997.

(© North Thames Regional Library and Information Unit 2001)

Appendix 2 – Some further sources of information and resources that facilitate evidence-based practice

BARBARA CUMBERS AND REINHARD WENTZ

Sources of systematic reviews

ACP Journal Club

(http://www.acponline.org/journals/acpjc/jcmenu.htm)
Published six times a year, ACP Journal Club is the critically acclaimed source to find the most important articles among the thousands published each year in peer-reviewed journals. ACP Journal Club's distinctive format facilitates rapid assessment of each study's validity and relevance to your clinical practice.

Bandolier

(http://www.jr2.ox.ac.uk/Bandolier)
Published monthly, available in printed format, and on the internet. Less rigorous than the others in this list, its reviews are in an easy-to-read style. The internet version is quickly and easily searchable. It has a broad though patchy coverage.

The Cochrane Library

http://www.update-software.com/cochrane/cochrane-frame.html (password necessary) or http://www.nelh.nhs.uk/cochrane.asp (password not necessary from an NHSnet connection). Updated quarterly. It is formed of several separate databases, including *The Cochrane Database of Systematic Reviews (CDSR)*, which contains the full text of specially compiled systematic reviews covering many branches of health care. It also contains the protocols and progress reports of systematic reviews that are currently being undertaken; *The Database of Abstracts of Reviews of Effectiveness (DARE)* which contains structured abstracts of good quality systematic reviews already published elsewhere; *The Cochrane Controlled Trials Register (CCTR)* which contains the bibliographic details and MEDLINE abstracts (if available) of trials identified as controlled. CCTR is by far the largest of the databases, by about two orders of magnitude. A search of the Cochrane Library searches all the databases, so search results will not all be systematic reviews. CDSR and DARE form part of EBMR on Ovid Biomed (with *ACP Journal Club*). The Cochrane Library is a good source to try first.

Effective Health Care

(http://www.york.ac.uk/inst/crd/ehcb.htm)
Published bi-monthly, these bulletins examine the effectiveness of a variety of health care interventions. Effective Health Care bulletins are based on systematic reviews and synthesis of research on the clinical effectiveness, cost-effectiveness and acceptability of health service interventions. This is carried out by a research team using established methodological guidelines, with advice from expert consultants for each topic. The bulletins are subject to extensive and rigorous peer review.

Effectiveness Matters

(http://www.york.ac.uk/inst/crd/em.htm)
Produced to complement Effective Health Care, it provides updates on the effectiveness of important health interventions for practitioners and decision makers in the NHS. It covers topics in a shorter and more journalistic style, summarising the results of high-quality systematic reviews. It is also subject to extensive and rigorous peer review.

Evidence-Based Medicine

(http://www.bmjpg.com/data/ebm.htm)
Available by subscription from the American College of Physicians and Canadian Medical Association and the BMJ Publishing Group, Specialist Journals Department, BMA House, Tavistock Square, London WC1H 9JR, UK (tel: + 44 171 387 4499). Published bi-monthly in printed format, and included with *ACP Journal Club* on a CD Rom called *Best Evidence*. Very similar in approach and format to *ACP Journal Club*, but covering general practice, surgery, psychiatry, paediatrics, obstetrics, and gynaecology.

NHS Centre for Reviews and Dissemination

(http://www.york.ac.uk/inst/crd/welcome.htm)
The NHS Centre for Reviews and Dissemination aims to identify and review the results of good quality health research and to disseminate the

findings to key decision makers in the NHS and to consumers of health care services. The reviews cover the effectiveness of care for particular conditions, the effectiveness of health technologies, and evidence on efficient methods of organising and delivering particular types of health care. Provides a more up-to-date version of *DARE* than the *Cochrane Library* (see above) as well as the *Economic Evaluations Database*.

Databases and search engines

PUBMED

(http://www.ncbi.nlm.nih.gov/entrez/query.fcgi)
Produced by the National Library of Medicine as their on-line version of MEDLINE. It is more up to date than other versions of MEDLINE, but very recent entries are often not indexed fully and do not contain abstracts. The "Clinical Queries" option (http://www.ncbi.nlm.nih.gov/entrez/query/static/clinical.html) provides the McMaster "methodological filters" (see pages 180–2) in an easy-to-use form.

SumSearch

(http://sumsearch.uthscsa.edu/searchform45.htm)
EBM-oriented search engine which searches Merck, DARE, PubMed, and other sources for relevant material and presents "hits" in a single document, arranged roughly by level of evidence.

TRIP database

(http://www.tripdatabase.com/)
A meta-search engine that searches across 61 sites of high-quality medical information, providing direct, hyperlinked access to the largest collection of databases of "evidence-based" material on the web as well as articles from premier on-line journals such as the *British Medical Journal, Journal of the American Medical Association* and *New England Journal of Medicine*. There are more than 15 000 links from these 61 sources; these are "evidence-based (direct links)", "evidence-based (indirect links)", "Peer-reviewed journals", "Guidelines" and finally "Other" (these tend to be textbook style entries that, while providing good quality information, may not be kept up to date)."). TRIP recently addded an "Extended Area" section to its sources, where EBHC-related material is grouped together by subjects.

Internet resources for evidence-based health care

CATbank.

(http://cebm.jr2.ox.ac.uk/docs/catbank.html)
A storage and retrieval facility for a collection of CATs (Critically Appraised Topics), developed by the Centre for Evidence-based Medicine to provide evidence-based answers to clinical problems.

Centre for Evidence-based Medicine

(http://cebm.jr2.ox.ac.uk)
The Centre for Evidence-based Medicine has been established in Oxford as the first of several centres around the UK whose aim broadly is to promote evidence-based health care and provide support and resources to anyone who wishes to make use of them.

The Cochrane Collaboration

(http://www.cochrane.org/)
Each Cochrane Centre throughout the world has its own website, through which others can be reached. The sites provide access to information on all Cochrane collaboration activities.

Evidence-based health

(http://www.mailbase.ac.uk/lists-a-e/evidence-based-health/)
A discussion list for teachers and practitioners in health-related fields to announce meetings and courses, stimulate discussion, air controversies, and aid the implementation of evidence-based health care.

National Electronic Library for Health (NeLH)

(http://www.nelh.nhs.uk/)
"The National Electronic Library for Health Programme is working with NHS Libraries to develop a digital library for NHS staff, patients, and the public. This is a pilot website (and the team welcome your feedback), aimed mainly at NHS staff. Patients, carers and the public are welcome to use this pilot, but NHS Direct Online provides the best public gateway to the library." A valuable source; its importance will grow and it is notable at the moment for providing free access (for NHS staff) to the full version of the **Cochrane Library** and **Clinical Evidence**. This is a site to watch. It also contains a "room" specifically for primary care staff at http://www.nelh-pc.nhs.uk/ where a "NeLH-PC Meta-Evidence Search Results" can be invoked.

Netting the Evidence – a ScHARR introduction to evidence-based practice on the internet

(http://www.shef.ac.uk/~scharr/ir/netting/
An alphabetical list of databases, journals, software, organisations, resources for searching for, appraising and implementing evidence, and a virtual library created by assembling links to full-text documents on all aspects of evidence-based practice.

Electronic guideline resources

Australian National Health and Medical Research Council (NHMRC)—full text versions of guidelines and other resources) (http://www.health. gov.au/nhmrc/publicat/cp-home.htm)

Canadian Medical Association Clinical Practice Guidelines Infobase—index of clinical practice guidelines, including downloadable full text versions or abstracts of most guidelines (http://www.cma. ca/cpgs/index.html)

CDC Prevention Guidelines Database a comprehensive compendium of all of the official guidelines and recommendations published by the US Centers for Disease Control and Prevention (CDC) for the prevention of diseases, injuries, and disabilities (http://aepo-xdv-www.epo.cdc.gov/wonder/prevguid/prevguid.htm)

Clinicians Health Channel Guidelines & Protocols (http://www.clinicians.vic.gov.au/guide.htm)

National Institute for Clinical Excellence—full text versions of guidelines and other resources (http://www.nice.org.uk)

New Zealand Guidelines Group—full text versions of guidelines and other resources (http://www.nzgg.org.nz/library.ctm)

Scottish Intercollegiate Guidelines Network—full text versions of guidelines and other resources (http://www.show.scot.nhs.uk/sign/graphic.htm)

US National Guidelines Clearing House—index of clinical guidelines including structured synopsis of development methods and key recommendations (http://www.guideline.gov/index.asp)

Additional resources

JAMA Users Guides to Evidence-based Practice
(http://www.cche.net/principles/content_all.asp)

Evidence-based medicine toolkit

(http://www.med.ualberta.ca/ebm/ebm.htm)

Critical Appraisal Skills Programme

(http://fester.his.path.cam.ac.uk/phealth/casphome.htm)

Critical Appraisal Skills Programme (CASP) is a UK project that aims to help health service decision makers develop skills in the critical appraisal of evidence about effectiveness, in order to promote the delivery of evidence-based health care. At the heart of CASP's work is a cascade of half-day workshops. These introduce participants to the key skills needed to find and make sense of evidence to support health service decisions, that is, CASP introduces people to the ideas of evidence-based medicine. Since workshops focus particularly on the critical appraisal of systematic reviews, CASP also introduces people to the related ideas of the Cochrane Collaboration.

Evidence-based care series

Setting priorities: how important is this problem? *Can Med Assoc J* 1994; **150**: 1249–54

Setting guidelines: how should we manage this problem? *Can Med Assoc J* 1994; **150**: 1417–23

Measuring performance: how are we managing this problem? *Can Med Assoc J* 1995; **150**: 1575–9

Improving performance: how are we improving the way we manage this problem? *Can Med Assoc J* 1994; **150**: 1793–6

Lifelong learning: how can we learn to be more effective? *Can Med Assoc J* 1994; **150**: 1971–3

Textbooks

Dixon RA, Munro JF, Silcocks PB. *The evidence-based medicine workbook. Critical appraisal for clinical problem solving.* Oxford: Butterworth-Heinemann, 1997

Dunn EV, Norton PG, Stewart M, Tudiver F, Bass MJ, eds. *Disseminating research/changing practice: research methods for primary care*, Vol 6. Thousand Oaks, CA: Sage, 1994

Gray JAM. *Evidence-based healthcare: how to make health policy and management decisions.* London: Churchill Livingstone, 1997.

Greenhalgh T. *How to read a paper. The basics of evidence-based medicine second edition.* London: BMJ Books, 2000

Haines A, Donald A. eds. *Getting research findings into practice second edition.* London, BMJ Books, 2001

Jones, R, Kinmonth A-L. eds. *Critical reading for primary care.* Oxford General Practice Series 28. Oxford: Oxford University Press, 1995

Panzer RJ, Black ER, Griner PE eds. *Diagnostic strategies for common medical problems*. Philadelphia: American College of Physicians, 1991

Rogers EM. *Diffusion of innovations*. New York: Free Press, 1983

Sackett DL, Haynes RB, Tugwell P. *Clinical epidemiology: a basic science for clinical medicine*. Boston/Toronto: Little, Brown, and Co. 1985

Sackett DL, Richardson SR, Rosenberg W, Haynes RB. *Evidence-based medicine: how to practice and teach EBM*. London: Churchill Livingstone, 1977

Index

Note: Page numbers in **bold** refer to figures; those in *italics* refer to tables and boxed material

Printed in the United Kingdom
by Lightning Source UK Ltd.
133926UK00002B/178-264/P